COVID-19: Impact on Public Health and Healthcare

COVID-19: Impact on Public Health and Healthcare

Approaches to Decrease the COVID-19 Impact

Editors

Manoj Sharma
Kavita Batra

MDPI • Basel • Beijing • Wuhan • Barcelona • Belgrade • Manchester • Tokyo • Cluj • Tianjin

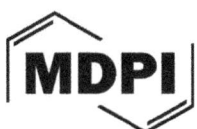

Editors
Manoj Sharma
Department of Social and
Behavioral Health
School of Public Health
University of Nevada, Las Vegas
USA

Kavita Batra
Office of Research, Kirk
Kerkorian School of Medicine
University of Nevada, Las Vegas
USA

Editorial Office
MDPI
St. Alban-Anlage 66
4052 Basel, Switzerland

This is a reprint of articles from the Topical Collection published online in the open access journal *Healthcare* (ISSN 2227-9032) (available at: https://www.mdpi.com/journal/healthcare/special_issues/covid-19_publichealth).

For citation purposes, cite each article independently as indicated on the article page online and as indicated below:

LastName, A.A.; LastName, B.B.; LastName, C.C. Article Title. *Journal Name* **Year**, *Volume Number*, Page Range.

ISBN 978-3-0365-2210-4 (Hbk)
ISBN 978-3-0365-2209-8 (PDF)

© 2021 by the authors. Articles in this book are Open Access and distributed under the Creative Commons Attribution (CC BY) license, which allows users to download, copy and build upon published articles, as long as the author and publisher are properly credited, which ensures maximum dissemination and a wider impact of our publications.

The book as a whole is distributed by MDPI under the terms and conditions of the Creative Commons license CC BY-NC-ND.

Contents

About the Editors . . . . **vii**

Preface to "COVID-19: Impact on Public Health and Healthcare" . . . . **ix**

Manoj Sharma, Kavita Batra, Robert E. Davis and Amanda H. Wilkerson
Explaining Handwashing Behavior in a Sample of College Students during COVID-19 Pandemic Using the Multi-Theory Model (MTM) of Health Behavior Change: A Single Institutional Cross-Sectional Survey
Reprinted from: *Healthcare* **2021**, *9*, 55, doi:10.3390/healthcare9010055 . . . . **1**

**Radomir Reszke, Marta Szepietowska, Piotr K. Krajewski, Łukasz Matusiak,
Rafał Białynicki-Birula and Jacek C. Szepietowski**
Face Mask Usage among Young Polish People during the COVID-19 Epidemic—
An Evolving Scenario
Reprinted from: *Healthcare* **2021**, *9*, 638, doi:10.3390/healthcare9060638 . . . . **17**

**Arnab Das, Adittya Barua, Md. Ajwad Mohimin, Jainal Abedin, Mayeen Uddin Khandaker
and Kholoud S. Al-mugren**
Development of a Novel Design and Subsequent Fabrication of an Automated Touchless Hand Sanitizer Dispenser to Reduce the Spread of Contagious Diseases
Reprinted from: *Healthcare* **2021**, *9*, 445, doi:10.3390/healthcare9040445 . . . . **29**

Kavita Batra, Yashashri Urankar, Ravi Batra, Aaron F. Gomes, Meru S and Pragati Kaurani
Knowledge, Protective Behaviors and Risk Perception of COVID-19 among Dental Students in India: A Cross-Sectional Analysis
Reprinted from: *Healthcare* **2021**, *9*, 574, doi:10.3390/healthcare9050574 . . . . **47**

**José F. Gómez-Clavel, Miguel A. Morales-Pérez, Gabriela Argumedo,
Cynthia G. Trejo-Iriarte and Alejandro García-Muñoz**
Concerns, Knowledge, and Practices of Dentists in Mexico Regarding Infection Control during the Coronavirus Disease Pandemic: A Cross-Sectional Study
Reprinted from: *Healthcare* **2021**, *9*, 731, doi:10.3390/healthcare9060731 . . . . **57**

**Gopi Battineni, Getu Gamo Sagaro, Nalini Chintalapudi, Marzio Di Canio and
Francesco Amenta**
Assessment of Awareness and Knowledge on Novel Coronavirus (COVID-19)
Pandemic among Seafarers
Reprinted from: *Healthcare* **2021**, *9*, 120, doi:10.3390/healthcare9020120 . . . . **69**

Xiaohan Zhang and Chao Wang
Prevention and Control of COVID-19 Pandemic on International Cruise Ships:
The Legal Controversies
Reprinted from: *Healthcare* **2021**, *9*, 281, doi:10.3390/healthcare9030281 . . . . **81**

Tsuyoshi Okuhara, Hiroko Okada and Takahiro Kiuchi
Predictors of Staying at Home during the COVID-19 Pandemic and Social Lockdown based on Protection Motivation Theory: A Cross-Sectional Study in Japan
Reprinted from: *Healthcare* **2020**, *8*, 475, doi:10.3390/healthcare8040475 . . . . **95**

Byungjin Park and Joonmo Cho
Older Adults' Avoidance of Public Transportation after the Outbreak of COVID-19:
Korean Subway Evidence
Reprinted from: *Healthcare* **2021**, *9*, 448, doi:10.3390/healthcare9040448 . . . . **107**

Manoj Sharma, Kavita Batra and Jason Flatt
Testing the Multi-Theory Model (MTM) to Predict the Use of New Technology for Social
Connectedness in the COVID-19 Pandemic
Reprinted from: *Healthcare* **2021**, *9*, 838, doi:10.3390/healthcare9070838 . . . . **123**

Da Hye Lee, Youn Su Kim, Young Youp Koh, Kwang Yoon Song and In Hong Chang
Forecasting COVID-19 Confirmed Cases Using Empirical Data Analysis in Korea
Reprinted from: *Healthcare* **2021**, *9*, 254, doi:10.3390/healthcare9030254 . . . . **139**

About the Editors

Manoj Sharma MBBS, Ph.D., MCHES® is currently a tenured Full Professor in the Department of Social and Behavioral Health at University of Nevada, Las Vegas in the School of Public Health. He is a prolific researcher and has published ten books, over 320 peer-reviewed research articles, and over 450 other publications and secured funding for over $5 million (h-index 41, i-10 index over 175, and over 9,000 citations). He has been awarded several prestigious honors including American Public Health Association's Mentoring Award, ICTHP Impact Award, and J. Mayhew. Derryberry Award, William R. Gemma Distinguished Alumnus Award from College of Public Health. Alumni Society (Ohio State University) and others. His research interests are in developing and evaluating theory-based health behavior change, obesity prevention, stress-coping, community-based participatory research, and integrative interventions.

Kavita Batra serves as a Biostatistician with the Nevada Department of Health and Human Services and the Kirk Kerkorian School of Medicine at UNLV. She provides statistical and research training to Medicine's faculty, residents, and fellows. Dr. Batra received her Ph.D. in Global and Environmental Health (GEH) from the University of Nevada, Las Vegas. Her research interests include but are not limited to maternal and child health, impact of COVID-19, and disparities among racial and gender minorities. Dr. Batra is an expert in qualitative and quantitative research and presented her work in several state and national public health conferences. She has published multiple peer reviewed articles to investigate the impact of COVID-19 on mental health and social connectedness across different demographic and workforce groups. Dr. Batra's recent work related to COVID-19 has been featured in reputed outlets, such as Medscape and Inside Higher Ed. Currently, she is editing three special issues.

Preface to "COVID-19: Impact on Public Health and Healthcare"

The sudden arrival of COVID-19 pandemic caused severe disruption in our lives. Initially, with no development of vaccines, preventive strategies, including social distancing, face mask wearing, handwashing, disinfection practices, and lockdown measures took precedence. These indirectly created issues of balance between public health interventions and individual rights. The lack of compliance towards preventive measures, insufficient knowledge about the transmission routes, and fear of contagion set a "perfect storm" for COVID-19 pandemic to take an aggressive form. The limited understanding about the COVID-19 pandemic triggered research in this area, which provided evidence for public health leaders and government agencies to design new programs and modify existing policies along the course of the pandemic.

This book aims to draw a comprehensive landscape of approaches utilized to reduce the far-ranging impacts of COVID-19 pandemic. Additionally, this compendium offers a diverse outlook of the preventive approaches to reduce COVID-19 transmission. The first two chapters in this book describe the preventive approaches, including handwashing behavior and facemask usage. Asian scientists from Bangladesh, Thailand, Malaysia, and Saudi Arabia describe a laser-based sensing sanitizer dispenser through an automated touchless process. The following two chapters describe protective behaviors and risk perceptions among dental staff, including doctors and students. Interestingly, awareness and knowledge about COVID-19 has also been investigated among Seafarers and legal controversies in the prevention/control of COVID-19 Pandemic on International Cruise Ships are explained in the next two chapters. Japanese researchers studied the predictors of staying home based on the Protection Motivation Theory. A group of Korean researchers investigated the avoidance of public transportation among older adults. Next study is about predicting the use of new technology to promote social connectedness during the COVID-19 pandemic using the fourth-generation multi-theory model (MTM) of health behavior change. Last chapter adds the useful dimensions of forecasting the COVID-19 burden for the effective control.

Manoj Sharma, Kavita Batra
Editors

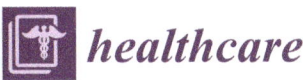

Article

Explaining Handwashing Behavior in a Sample of College Students during COVID-19 Pandemic Using the Multi-Theory Model (MTM) of Health Behavior Change: A Single Institutional Cross-Sectional Survey

Manoj Sharma [1], Kavita Batra [2,*], Robert E. Davis [3] and Amanda H. Wilkerson [4]

[1] Department of Environmental and Occupational Health, University of Nevada, Las Vegas, NV 89119, USA; manoj.sharma@unlv.edu
[2] Office of Research, School of Medicine, University of Nevada, Las Vegas, NV 89102, USA
[3] Substance Use and Mental Health Laboratory, Department of Health, Human Performance and Recreation, University of Arkansas, Fayetteville, AR 72701, USA; red007@uark.edu
[4] Human Environmental Sciences, University of Alabama, Tuscaloosa, AL 35487, USA; awilkerson@ches.ua.edu
* Correspondence: kavita.batra@unlv.edu; Tel.: +1-702-895-2655

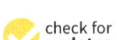

Citation: Sharma, M.; Batra, K.; Davis, R.E.; Wilkerson, A.H. Explaining Handwashing Behavior in a Sample of College Students during COVID-19 Pandemic Using the Multi-Theory Model (MTM) of Health Behavior Change: A Single Institutional Cross-Sectional Survey. *Healthcare* **2021**, *9*, 55. https://doi.org/10.3390/healthcare9010055

Received: 20 November 2020
Accepted: 3 January 2021
Published: 6 January 2021

Publisher's Note: MDPI stays neutral with regard to jurisdictional claims in published maps and institutional affiliations.

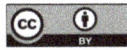

Copyright: © 2021 by the authors. Licensee MDPI, Basel, Switzerland. This article is an open access article distributed under the terms and conditions of the Creative Commons Attribution (CC BY) license (https://creativecommons.org/licenses/by/4.0/).

Abstract: Amidst the COVID-19 pandemic, handwashing offers a simple and effective hygienic measure for disease prevention. Reportedly, a significant proportion of college students did not follow handwashing recommendations provided by the Centers for Disease Control and Prevention (CDC) in the pre-COVID era. The purpose of this cross-sectional study was to explore and explain the handwashing behavior among college students during the COVID-19 pandemic using a contemporary fourth-generation multi-theory model (MTM) of health behavior change. Data were collected from 713 college students at a large public university in the Southern U.S. in October 2020 using a validated 36-item survey. Statistical analyses included independent samples t-tests, Pearson correlation, and hierarchical regression modeling. Among students not following handwashing recommendations, the constructs of participatory dialogue ($\beta = 0.152$; $p < 0.05$) and behavioral confidence ($\beta = 0.474$; $p < 0.0001$) were statistically significant and accounted for 27.2% of the variance in the likelihood of initiation of the behavior. Additionally, the constructs of emotional transformation ($\beta = 0.330$; $p < 0.0001$), practice for change ($\beta = 0.296$; $p < 0.0001$), and changes in the social environment ($\beta = 0.180$; $p < 0.05$) were statistically significant and accounted for 45.1% of the variance in the likelihood of sustaining handwashing behavior. This study highlights the applicability and usability of the MTM in designing and testing behavior change interventions and media messaging in campaigns targeting college students.

Keywords: multi-theory model; behavior change; COVID-19; pandemic; handwashing; young adults; college students

1. Introduction

The novel coronavirus (COVID-19) disease caused by the SARS-CoV-2 virus has rapidly spiraled across the world and took the course of pandemic [1,2]. As of 18 November 2020, there are a total of 55,064,128 confirmed cases and 1,328,015 deaths attributable to COVID-19 worldwide, with a sizable proportion reported in the United States alone [2,3]. To reduce the spread of COVID-19, public health officials have encouraged various safety and mitigation strategies, including hygiene measures, such as handwashing, sneezing into an elbow, avoiding touching surfaces, and wearing personal protective equipment [1].

One of the simple yet effective measures recommended by the government and public health agencies is frequent and thorough handwashing [4,5]. Handwashing is a longstanding, non-pharmacologic public health measure, which has proven to minimize the spread of gastrointestinal and respiratory infections by 31% and 21%, respectively [6,7]. Handwashing removes microorganisms from the hands and prevents their transfer through different media, such as foods, beverages, and inanimate objects [8]. The CDC recommends scrubbing hands thoroughly with soap and water for at least 20 s under running water and drying hands with a clean towel or air drying for effective hand cleaning [4,8]. The CDC encourages public to wash their hands at a minimum during the following circumstances: (1) after being in public; (2) before and after providing care for someone who is sick; (3) after blowing their nose, sneezing, or coughing; (4) before, during, and after food preparation; (5) before eating food; (6) after using the toilet; (7) after touching an animal; and (8) after touching garbage [4,8].

College campuses and their surrounding communities became a central concern for COVID-19 prevention due to surging trends of COVID-19 among young adults aged 20–29 in the U.S. since June 2020 [9,10]. The CDC and American College Health Association published guidelines and considerations for reopening campuses amid the pandemic, including recommendations to emphasize hand hygiene practices on campus [8,11]. Research in the pre-COVID-19 era reported a lack of adherence or compliance to the handwashing regimen among college student and university community samples [12–14]. The rate of compliance varied from 38.5% to 66.9%, which underscores the need for interventions to promote handwashing behavior in this group [12–14]. Previous theory-based interventions successfully promoted good handwashing practices among young adults [15–17]. However, more research is needed to reinforce and sustain these handwashing practices among college students at the time of COVID-19 crisis, while the development of pharmacologic interventions is underway.

Recent studies reported that female students and those with the positive attitudes and knowledge towards handwashing for COVID-19 prevention were more likely to adopt handwashing behavior [18,19]. Further, studies utilized the theory of planned behavior, health action process approach, and health belief model to explain handwashing behavior in college students and adults during the COVID-19 pandemic [20]. Positive attitudes, positive subjective norms about handwashing behavior, higher perceived benefits of handwashing, and lower barriers to handwashing were associated with adherence to proper handwashing [20]. Additional information on factors related to initiation and continuation of the handwashing behavior to prevent COVID-19 spread is needed to ensure greater behavior adoption rates among college students.

The current study uses a contemporary, fourth-generation theoretical framework, the multi-theory model (MTM) for health behavior change, to explore handwashing behavior among college students. The MTM is a health behavior change theory with the unique ability to explain factors related to one-time (e.g., initiation) and long-term (e.g., sustenance) engagement in health behavior [21]. The constructs are adaptable across health behaviors and have been used to explain a variety of health behaviors among college students [22–27]). For initiation, the MTM posits that participatory dialogue (i.e., advantages counterweighing disadvantages of handwashing), behavioral confidence (i.e., a sureness in properly following steps of thorough handwashing despite obstacles), and changes in the physical environment (i.e., availability and accessibility of necessary resources for handwashing) will be instrumental in behavior change [21,28–30]. Whereas, for sustenance, emotional transformation (i.e., converting feelings into goals for regular handwashing), practice for change (i.e., creating a habit of handwashing and making it a way of life), and changes in the social environment (i.e., fostering social support from the environment) are important for long-term adherence to the changed behaviors [21,30,31].

Previous health behavior theoretical models focused on behavior acquisition rather than change have yielded mixed results when exploring behavior change, are documented to lack substantive predictive power, and are not suited to determine long-term behavior change [21]. The MTM is a unique theoretical framework due to identifying antecedents for both initiation and sustenance of behavior. Identifying factors related to the initiation and sustenance of handwashing using the MTM can inform the development of handwashing interventions for college students in the short and long term. Therefore, the study aimed to explain handwashing behavior during the COVID-19 pandemic among college students using the MTM. The findings of this study can be utilized to develop effective health promotion interventions to encourage handwashing behavior for this target audience.

2. Materials and Methods

2.1. Study Design and Study Participants

This descriptive, quantitative, cross-sectional survey study was conducted from 8 October 2020, to 29 October 2020, among college students at a large public Southern US university. The survey was deemed the most appropriate design due to its inherent capacity to collect information with relative ease from large population groups within a given period [32]. Students currently enrolled in any university programs, who were aged 18 years or above, had internet access, could provide informed consent, and comprehend English, were invited to participate in this survey. Alumni and those with no Internet access and an inability to understand English were excluded from this study.

2.2. Ethical Considerations

This study followed the Checklist for Reporting Results of Internet E-Surveys (CHERRIES) guidelines [33]. This study was deemed exempt from the university's institutional review board (Protocol # 2009281493) on 21 September 2020. All participants were requested to provide their informed consent by answering an agree/disagree question, thereby confirming their willingness to participate. Informed consent included detailed information related to the study's aim and significance and informed participants of their right to withdraw at any point. Participants who selected the "agree" option were directed to complete an online questionnaire. Personal identifiers, including names, email I.D.s, and details of COVID-19 exposure, were not collected. Only one response per I.P. address was allowed.

2.3. Recruitment and Data Collection

The convenience sampling method was used for sample recruitment. Participants were recruited through advertisements posted on the university's daily e-news bulletin, intended to disseminate information to faculty, students, and staff with a valid university email address. The recruitment advertisement containing an anonymous survey link with complete details of the study was sent out every Thursday for three consecutive weeks to all currently enrolled students (27,562). Upon clicking the link, interested participants were connected to the Qualtrics (Provo, UT) interface to access and fill out the web-based survey. As an incentive, participants were informed that by participating, they had the opportunity to enter a drawing to win one of five $20.00 Walmart gift cards. The final survey item asked students about their willingness to enter the drawing to receive one of the gift cards. Interested students clicked 'yes', which functioned as a link to a separate survey where an email address could be collected for contact purposes. This process preserved participant anonymity by making it impossible to link the provided email address to data previously disclosed during the data collection process. The Qualtrics survey options were set to prevent "ballot box stuffing." This option restricts the same IP address from contributing in multiple surveys. Participants who accessed the survey link more than once would receive a message that their responses had already been recorded.

2.4. Survey Instrument

Handwashing encompasses five steps from wetting the hands with running water, applying lather by rubbing soap, scrubbing hands thoroughly for at least 20 s, rinsing hands under running water, followed by drying with a clean towel or air drying them [34]. Utilizing the MTM theoretical framework, a survey instrument to assess the likelihood of initiating and sustaining handwashing behavior was developed. The instrument consisted of 36 items with six items related to participant demography. The remaining 30 items correspond to two main components of the MTM, such as initiation and sustenance, with a total of seven constructs. In the initiation, the first construct is participatory dialogue measuring advantages (five items) and disadvantages (five items) of handwashing behavior on a 5-point scale from never (0) to very often (5). The possible score ranges of advantages and disadvantages were 0–20, with a high score on advantages and a low score on disadvantages depicting the likelihood of the behavior change. The score of the participatory dialogue was computed after deducting the disadvantages score from the advantages score. The score range of participatory dialogue varies from −24 to +24 units [35]. The second construct of initiation was behavioral confidence, which implies confidence in making the behavior change with external or internal driving sources [35]. Behavioral confidence measured the likelihood of initiation of behavior change with six items and a score ranging from 0 to 24 [35]. Another construct of initiation was "changes in the physical environment," which encompasses alterations related to the accessibility of resources or factors to initiate behavior change [35]. The physical environment change was assessed on three items, and the score ranges from 0–12 units.

The second element of MTM: sustenance has three constructs, namely emotional transformation (converting emotions to the goals), practice for change (self-assessment, overcoming barriers, focused on consistency with the behavior change), and changes in the social environment (support from the social circle for the behavior change). These constructs were measured using three items, each with a score range of 0–12 units [35]. The instrument used clear and appropriate language, which corresponds to the Flesch reading ease of 69.6 and Flesch–Kincaid Grade Level of fifth grade [36]. A panel of six subject matter, instrumentation, and target group experts assessed the instrument's face and content validity and provided feedback. The instrument was advanced to the second round after addressing the feedback (16 modifications were made) before the finalization of the tool.

2.5. Statistical Analyses

Participants' responses from Qualtrics^{XM} were exported to Microsoft Excel (Microsoft Corporation, Richmond VA, USA) and then imported to IBM SPSS version 26.0 (IBM Corp. Armonk NY, USA). Confirmatory factor analysis using the maximum likelihood method and internal consistency diagnostic tests using Cronbach's alpha were performed to check the construct validity and internal consistency of the tool. For establishing a one-factor solution following the Kaiser criterion of Eigenvalue greater than or equal to 1.0, factor loadings on each item greater than 0.326 (after doubling the critical value for a sample size of 250 at an $\alpha = 0.01$ for a two-tailed test) were established a priori as per the generally accepted recommendations from previous literature [36–38]. For establishing internal consistency reliability, a Cronbach's alpha of ≥ 0.70 was considered acceptable [36]. Descriptive statistics, including the frequencies, proportions, mean, and standard deviations, were generated. The likelihood of intention and sustenance of handwashing behavior were the dependent variables, while the constructs were used as independent variables. To analyze the differences in mean scores across different groups who follow or did not follow handwashing recommendations, an independent-samples t-test was utilized. Pearson's correlations test was utilized to calculate correlations among the variables. p-values less than 0.05 (two-sided) were considered statistically significant, and data were reported with 95% confidence intervals. Hierarchical multiple regression was utilized to predict the likelihood of initiation and sustenance of handwashing behavior based on multiple regressors or independent variables, such as age, gender, race/ethnicity, and individual constructs of the MTM. Gender and race/ethnicity variables were dummy coded. Assumptions of independence of observations (i.e., Durbin–Watson statistic), linearity (e.g., scatterplot and partial regression plots), homoscedasticity, multicollinearity, and normality (1.e., P-P plot and Q-Q plot) were evaluated on the full model.

2.6. Sample Size Justification

G*power software (version 3.1) was used to perform a priori power analysis [39]. The a priori power analysis was conducted to ascertain the required sample size for a test with a predetermined alpha and beta (power) level. For multiple regression, the alpha was set at 0.05, power at 0.80, five predictors (three MTM constructs and three covariates), and the effect size at 0.06 (small to medium), and this yielded a sample size of 234. After factoring in 10% incomplete entries or missing values, our minimum sample requirement was 257 (234 + 23 = 257).

3. Results

3.1. Sample Characteristics

A total of 713 valid responses were recorded during the survey period. The demographic profile of the respondent's shows that 501 (70.3%) respondents identified as females and 176 (24.7%) were males (Table 1). The average age of the sample was 24.61 years (SD = 8.60 years). Nearly three-fourths of the participants were white (74.3%, n = 503) (Table 1). Most of the participants were undergraduate students (67.7%, n = 483), with nearly one-fourth (n = 197) being enrolled in the graduate program (Table 1). Further, 68.6% of students reported washing their hands at least six times over the past day (Table 1).

Table 1. Descriptive statistics of the demographic variables of the study population (n = 713).

Variable	Characteristics	Mean ± S.D.	n (%)
Age	-	24.61 ± 8.60	-
Gender	Female	-	501 (70.3)
	Male	-	176 (24.7)
	Others	-	14 (2.0)
	Not reported	-	22 (3.1)
Race/ethnicity	White/Caucasian	-	530 (74.3)
	Black or African	-	33 (4.6)
	Hispanic or Latino	-	56 (7.9)
	Asian American	-	39 (5.4)
	Others	-	31 (4.4)
	Not reported	-	24 (3.4)
Current year in school	First-year undergraduate	-	164 (23.0)
	Second-year undergraduate	-	95 (13.3)
	Third-year undergraduate	-	90 (12.6)
	Fourth-year undergraduate	-	104 (14.6)
	Fifth-year undergraduate	-	30 (4.2)
	Graduate	-	195 (27.3)
	Professional degree	-	11 (1.5)
	Not reported	-	24 (3.4)
Employment	Yes	-	373 (52.3)
	No	-	318 (44.6)
	Not reported	-	22 (3.1)
Number of hours worked weekly *	-	23.0 ± 12.3	-
Hand washing at least six times in the past day	Yes	-	489 (68.6)
	No	-	224 (31.4)

* Numbers of hours were reported by 340 (47.7%) participants only.

3.2. Characteristics of Study Variables and Inferential Statistics

Construct validation revealed a one-factor solution for each subscale and Eigenvalues greater than 1. All factor loadings were over the critical value of 0.326. The Cronbach's alpha for all subscales was at least 0.70 (lowest = 0.70; highest = 0.96; Table 2) and were deemed acceptable [36].

There were significant differences in mean scores of initiation and sustenance across groups following or not following handwashing recommendations (Table 2). The mean initiation score was higher among those following handwashing recommendations (M = 3.40, SD = 0.88) than those not following (M = 2.3, SD = 1.14), with a statistically significant mean difference, M = 1.1, 95% CI [1.01, 1.29], $p < 0.0001$, Table 2). Similarly, the mean score of sustenance was higher (M = 3.35, SD = 0.90) following handwashing recommendations than those not following (M = 2.16, SD = 1.13), with a statistically significant mean difference, M = 1.2, 95% CI [1.01, 1.4], $p < 0.0001$, Table 2). The likelihood of initiation and sustenance was significantly correlated with all the constructs, at 0.01 levels of significance, for both groups (Table 3).

Hierarchical multiple regression was run to determine if the sequential addition of participatory dialogue, changes in the physical environment, and behavioral confidence improved the likelihood of initiation over and above demographic variables (Table 4). Among participants following handwashing recommendations, the full model (Model 4) to predict initiation was statistically significant, $R^2 = 0.479$, $F (6, 406) = 62.157$, $p < 0.0001$; adjusted $R^2 = 0.471$ (Table 4). The addition of participatory dialogue to the prediction of initiation (Model 2) led to a statistically significant increase in R^2 of 0.240, $F (1, 408) = 130.32$, $p < 0.0001$. The addition of behavioral confidence to the prediction of initiation (Model 3) led to a statistically significant increase in R^2 of 0.222, $F (1407) = 170.97$, $p < 0.0001$.

In the hierarchical regression with sustenance as the dependent variable, the full model (Model 4) was statistically significant, $R^2 = 0.434$, $F (6, 415) = 52.953$, $p < 0.0001$; adjusted $R^2 = 0.425$ (Table 4). The addition of emotional transformation to the prediction of sustenance (Model 2) led to a statistically significant increase in R^2 of 0.372, $F (1, 417) = 255.710$, $p < 0.0001$. The addition of practice for change to the prediction of sustenance (Model 3) led to a statistically significant increase in R^2 of 0.038, $F (1, 416) = 27.413$, $p < 0.0001$.

Among participants not following handwashing recommendations, the full model (Model 4) to predict initiation was statistically significant, $R^2 = 0.295$, $F (6, 181) = 12.615$, $p < 0.0001$; adjusted $R^2 = 0.272$ (Table 5). The addition of behavior confidence to the prediction of initiation (Model 3) led to a statistically significant increase in R^2 of 0.162, $F (1, 182) = 41.784$, $p < 0.0001$ (Table 5). The addition of participatory dialogue to the prediction of initiation (Model 2) also led to a statistically significant increase in R^2 of 0.117, $F (1, 183) = 24.682$, $p < 0.0001$. In the hierarchical regression with sustenance as a dependent variable, the full model (Model 4) was statistically significant, $R^2 = 0.468$, $F (6184) = 26.972$, $p < 0.0001$; adjusted $R^2 = 0.451$ (Table 5).The addition of emotional transformation to the prediction of sustenance (Model 2) led to a statistically significant increase in R^2 of 0.344, $F (1, 186) = 100.790$, $p < 0.0001$. The addition of practice for change to the prediction of sustenance (Model 3) led to a statistically significant increase in R^2 of 0.080, $F (1, 185) = 26.772$, $p < 0.0001$. The addition of changes in the social environment to the prediction of sustenance (Model 4) led to a statistically significant increase in R^2 of 0.023, F (1, 184) = 7.957, $p < 0.05$.

Table 2. Descriptive statistics of multi-theory model constructs of behavior change (n = 713) and reliability diagnostics.

Groups	Those Who Followed Handwashing Recommendations (n = 489)				Those Who Did Not Follow Handwashing Recommendations (n = 224)				
Constructs	Possible score range	Observed score range	Mean ± S.D.	Cronbach's alpha	Possible score range	Observed score range	Mean ± S.D.	Cronbach's alpha	p-value
Initiation	0–4	0–4	3.40 ± 0.88	-	0–4	0–4	2.3 ± 1.14	-	<0.0001
Participatory dialogue: advantages	0–20	0–20	16.40 ± 4.85	0.96	0–20	0–20	15.24 ± 5.35	0.96	0.004
Participatory dialogue: disadvantages	0–20	0–20	4.35±3.73	0.81	0–20	0–17	7.21 ± 4.13	0.74	<0.0001
Participatory dialogue: advantages—disadvantages score	−20–20	−20–20	12.75 ± 6.25	-	−20–+20	−13–+20	9.13 ± 6.14	-	<0.0001
Behavioral confidence	0–24	4–24	20.12 ± 4.41	0.90	0–24	0–24	15.9 ± 5.3	0.87	<0.0001
Changes in the physical environment	0–12	0–12	10.52 ± 2.1	0.83	0–12	2–12	9.7 ± 2.52	0.78	<0.0001
Entire initiation scale	-	-	-	0.72	-	-	-	0.69	-
Sustenance	0–4	0–4	3.35 ± 0.90	-	0–4	0–4	2.16 ± 1.13	-	<0.0001
Emotional transformation	0–12	1–12	9.85 ± 2.5	0.88	0–12	0–12	7.34 ± 3.04	0.87	<0.0001
Practice for change	0–12	0–12	7.96 ± 2.75	0.70	0–12	0–12	5.4 ± 2.73	0.76	<0.0001
Changes in the social environment	0–12	0–12	7.35 ± 3.74	0.87	0–12	0–12	4.43 ± 3.82	0.85	<0.0001
Entire sustenance scale	-	-	-	0.88	-	-	-	0.87	-
Entire scale	-	-	-	0.86	-	-	-	0.85	-

Table 3. Correlation matrix of the initiation and sustenance model constructs.

	Construct(s)	1	2	3	4
	Those who followed handwashing recommendations (n = 489)				
1	Likelihood for Initiation	-	0.358 **	0.671 **	0.515 **
2	Participatory dialogue: advantages—disadvantages score	-	-	0.464 **	0.365 **
3	Behavioral confidence	-	-	-	0.631 **
4	Changes in the physical environment	-	-	-	-
1	Likelihood for Sustenance	-	0.625 **	0.550 **	0.378 **
2	Emotional Transformation	-	-	0.651 **	0.418 **
3	Practice for Change	-	-	-	0.565 **
4	Changes in the Social Environment	-	-	-	-
	Those who did not follow handwashing recommendations (n = 224)	1	2	3	4
1	Likelihood for Initiation	-	0.361 **	0.520 **	0.284 **
2	Participatory dialogue: advantages—disadvantages score	-	-	0.469 **	0.483 **
3	Behavioral confidence	-	-	-	0.537 **
4	Changes in the physical environment	-	-	-	-
1	Likelihood for Sustenance	-	0.602 **	0.604 **	0.476 **
2	Emotional Transformation	-	-	0.643 **	0.423 **
3	Practice for Change	-	-	-	0.516 **
4	Changes in the Social Environment	-	-	-	-

** p values are significant <0.01.

Table 4. Hierarchical multiple regression predicting likelihood for initiation and sustenance of handwashing behavior among respondents following recommendations (n = 489).

Variables	Model 1 B	Model 1 β	Model 2 B	Model 2 β	Model 3 B	Model 3 β	Model 4 B	Model 4 β
	\multicolumn{8}{c}{The likelihood for initiation as a dependent variable}							
Constant	3.334 **		2.386 **		0.874 **		0.629 **	
Age	0.001	0.008	0.001	0.008	−0.006	−0.057	−0.005	−0.050
Gender	−0.141	−0.080	−0.004	−0.002	0.027	0.015	0.027	0.015
Race/Ethnicity	0.106	0.054	0.132	0.066	0.056	0.028	0.045	0.023
Participatory dialogue			0.070 **	0.496	0.022 **	0.159	0.019 *	0.137
Behavioral confidence					0.116 **	0.585	0.104 **	0.524
Changes in the physical environment							0.049*	0.116
R^2	0.009		0.249		0.471		0.479	
F	1.256		33.819 **		72.520 **		62.157 **	
ΔR^2	0.009		0.240		0.222		0.008	
ΔF^2	1.256		130.318 **		170.971 **		5.940 *	
	\multicolumn{8}{c}{The likelihood for sustenance as a dependent variable}							
Constant	3.231 **		1.282 **		1.256 **		1.254 **	
Age	0.007	0.071	−0.003	−0.026	−0.006	−0.058	−0.007	−0.062
Gender	−0.240 *	−0.133	−0.061	−0.034	−0.036	−0.020	−0.034	−0.019
Race/ethnicity	−0.003	−0.002	−0.044	−0.022	−0.052	−0.026	−0.051	−0.026
Emotional transformation			0.222 **	0.624	0.164 **	0.461	0.162 **	0.456
Practice for change					0.085 **	0.259	0.073 **	0.224
Changes in the social environment							0.017	0.070
R^2	0.020		0.393		0.430		0.434	
F	2.901 *		67.430 **		62.843 **		52.953 **	
ΔR^2	0.020		0.372		0.038		0.003	
ΔF^2	2.901 *		255.71 **		27.41 **		2.	

B (Unstandardized coefficient); β (Standardized coefficient), * p-value < 0.05; ** p-value < 0.001; Adjusted R^2 of initiation = 0.471; Adjusted R^2 of sustenance = 0.425.

Table 5. Hierarchical multiple regression predicting likelihood for initiation and sustenance of handwashing behavior among respondents not following recommendations (n = 224).

Variables	Model 1 B	Model 1 β	Model 2 B	Model 2 β	Model 3 B	Model 3 β	Model 4 B	Model 4 β
The likelihood for initiation as a dependent variable								
Constant	2.563 **		1.852 **		0.684 *		0.771 *	
Age	−0.005	−0.042	−0.003	−0.022	0.000	−0.003	−0.001	−0.004
Gender	−0.234	−0.028	−0.057	−0.026	−0.015	−0.007	−0.014	−0.007
Race/ethnicity	−0.075	−0.028	−0.069	−0.026	−0.206	−0.078	−0.197	−0.074
Participatory dialogue			0.065 **	0.352	0.026 **	0.142	0.028 *	0.152
Behavioral confidence					0.099 **	0.461	0.102 **	0.474
Changes in the physical environment							−0.016	−0.035
R^2	0.015		0.132		0.294		0.295	
F	0.931		6.959 **		15.164 **		12.615 **	
ΔR^2	0.015		0.117		0.162		0.001	
ΔF^2	0.931		24.682 **		41.784 **		0.202	
The likelihood for sustenance as a dependent variable								
Constant	2.533 **		0.700 *		0.525		0.481	
Age	−0.007	−0.060	−0.003	−0.027	−0.003	−0.021	−0.001	−0.011
Gender	−0.246	−0.113	−0.033	−0.015	−0.047	−0.022	−0.059	−0.027
Race/ethnicity	−0.128	−0.049	−0.086	−0.033	−0.098	−0.037	−0.064	−0.024
Emotional transformation			0.222 **	0.597	0.133 **	0.358	0.122 **	0.330
Practice for change					0.154 **	0.370	0.123 **	0.296
Changes in the social environment							0.053 *	0.180
R^2	0.020		0.365		0.445		0.468	
F	1.293		26.685 **		29.660 **		26.972 **	
ΔR^2	0.020		0.344		0.080		0.023	
ΔF^2	1.293		100.790 **		26.772 **		7.957 *	

B (Unstandardized coefficient); β (Standardized coefficient), * p-value < 0.05; ** p-value < 0.01; Adjusted R^2 of initiation = 0.272; Adjusted R^2 of sustenance = 0.451.

4. Discussion

The study utilized the MTM, a novel fourth-generation behavioral theory, to explain handwashing behavior among college students during the COVID-19 pandemic. Despite the aggressive media messages and recommendations from governmental authorities, the study revealed that 31.4% of the college students did not practice frequent handwashing in the recommended manner compared to 33.1% to 61.5% reported in pre-COVID-19 era [12–14]. This study shows that the proportion of young adults not following the handwashing guidelines remains a matter of concern in these times. This finding points to the urgent need to design individual-level behavior change educational interventions and community-level media campaigns directed specifically toward this subgroup to mitigate the COVID-19 transmission.

This study revealed that approximately 27.2% of the variance in the likelihood to practice initiation was significantly predicted by behavioral confidence (i.e., a sureness in properly following steps of thorough handwashing despite barriers) and participatory dialogue (i.e., assessing advantages and disadvantages of handwashing), among those not following the handwashing recommendations ($p < 0.0001$). Participatory dialogue will be higher in the magnitude if advantages outweigh disadvantages and will be lower in the reverse scenario. This can be validated by the participatory dialogue score among students not following the handwashing recommendations, who perceive handwashing having more disadvantages than advantages. Every unit increase in behavioral confidence resulted in a 0.474 unit increase in the likelihood of the initiation of handwashing behavior. Similarly, for every unit increase in participatory dialogue, a 0.152 increase in the likelihood of the initiation of handwashing behavior ensued. Among students following the handwashing recommendations ($n = 489$, Table 4), all three constructs of initiation are statistically significant and account for approximately 47.1% of the variance in the response variable. The magnitude of these associations, as represented by adjusted R^2, is considered substantial in behavioral and social science research [36]. Similar to behavioral confidence, a construct of self-efficacy has adequately been used to reinforce handwashing behavior among general populations [40–43]. The statistical significance of participatory dialogue and behavioral confidence has already been established in studying other behaviors (intake of sweetened beverages, binge drinking, portion size consumption, fruits, and vegetable consumption, and intentional outdoor nature contact) among college students [22–27,44,45].

Further, it is worth noting that significant differences between all three initiation constructs in the MTM for initiation were statistically significant ($p < 0.0001$) and greater among those who were practicing the recommendations for handwashing compared to those who were not. This finding lends support to the predictability of MTM for the initiation of handwashing behavior among college students. Future research and individual-level behavior change interventions and media campaigns should utilize the constructs of participatory dialogue and behavioral confidence in promoting handwashing behavior among college students.

Regarding the MTM's ability to predict maintaining handwashing behavior, the examination of the sustenance model among those not following the recommendations revealed 45.1% of the variance in the likelihood to continue the practice of handwashing. Additionally, sustenance significantly predicted by all three constructs: emotional transformation (i.e., converting feelings into goals of regular handwashing) ($p < 0.0001$), practice for change (i.e., creating a habit of handwashing and making it a way of life) ($p < 0.0001$), and changes in the social environment (i.e., fostering social support from the environment) ($p < 0.05$). For every unit increase in emotional transformation, there is a 0.33 unit increase in the likelihood of maintaining handwashing behavior; for every unit increase in practice for change construct, there is a 0.296 increase in the likelihood of maintaining handwashing behavior; and for every unit increase in the changes in the social environment score, there is a 0.180 increase in the likelihood of maintaining handwashing behavior. The findings are also supported by data of students practicing handwashing according to recommendations ($n = 489$, Table 4), in which emotional transformation and practice for change are statistically significant and account for approximately 42.5% of the variance in the likelihood of sustaining handwashing behavior. Furthermore, the differences between all the three constructs of MTM for sustenance were statistically significant ($p < 0.0001$) and higher among those who were practicing the recommendations for handwashing as compared to those who were not, which further lends support to the predictive potential of MTM for the sustenance of handwashing behavior among college students.

Emotional transformation (i.e., converting feelings into goals) plays an important role in the sustenance of a behavior [21,35,46–49]. The construct of emotional transformation has also been found to be a statistically significant construct in other studies done among college students with other behaviors [22,24,26,27,44,45]. Individual-level behavior change interventions and media campaigns for college students must be designed to appeal to their emotions and get them toward concrete goals of handwashing behavior. Among studies conducted with non-college student populations, there is limited evidence of changes in the social environment or social support about maintaining handwashing behavior [41,50]. However, similar to previous constructs, the construct of changes in the social environment also derives backing from studies with other behaviors, such as sleep, eating, and drinking behaviors that have been done among college students [22,24,26,27,44,45]. Therefore, the importance of these constructs to the maintenance of handwashing behavior is also justified.

4.1. Implications for Practice

The study has important implications for designing handwashing promotion interventions, especially during the COVID-19 pandemic. The findings point to the fact that, despite the pandemic mounting at alarming rates, a substantial proportion of college students do not wash their hands as per the CDC recommendations. This issue can be addressed by designing individual-level behavioral change educational interventions and media campaigns (i.e., including social media) directed toward college students. Individual-level behavior change interventions can be delivered through classrooms or other university channels using the learning management systems (LMS) such as Blackboard, Canvas, Moodle, Brightspace, which almost all universities utilize to access course content. Further, as a policy measure supportive of behavior change, such interventions can be mandated by the university administration.

MTM has been used in designing similar technology-based brief and specific interventions [51–53] and can be effectively used for handwashing promotion among college students. The construct of participatory dialogue, which is quite intuitive and points to the underscoring the advantages of handwashing over any possible disadvantages, can be built by effective tailored messaging. Messages such as, "Handwashing is cool," "Handwashing makes hands smell good," and "Handwashing makes you attractive" can be used on both an individual level as well as media campaigns. Social media sites such as Facebook, Instagram, WhatsApp, and Twitter can be mobilized to promote these messages. Behavioral confidence can be built by demonstrating handwashing through videos that show the handwashing process in small steps. Additionally, potential barriers can be addressed by tailored messages such as making time to wash hands, having reminder messages, and overcoming inconvenience. These messages can be incorporated into the public health educational campaigns along with the standard guidelines of the regulatory agencies. Physical barriers, such as readily available water supply and soap, did not emerge as a significant factor in this U.S. sample but may be necessary for resource-constrained low and middle-income countries for which appropriate policy measures should be considered.

Concerning sustenance constructs, emotional transformation emerged as the most influential construct in this study, and the importance of channeling one's feelings cannot be overemphasized. To build this construct, the first step is to be cognizant of one's feelings, which is vital in changing handwashing behavior and changing any behavior and self-improvement [31]. After identifying feelings, especially negative ones, individuals should be directed toward establishing goals. In the case of handwashing promotion interventions, the goal should be to wash hands frequently in the recommended manner until it becomes second nature. The construct of practice for change can be built by teaching college students to self-reflect and self-monitor their handwashing behavior. Finally, the support of family, friends, peers, instructors, health professionals, and other significant influences must be emphasized in handwashing promotion interventions.

4.2. Strengths and Limitations of the Study

To our knowledge, this study is among the very few theory-based or evidence-based studies that have been performed on handwashing behavior among college students during the COVID-19 pandemic. This study offers a unique perspective by utilizing newer multiple theory models for studying handwashing behavior among college students. Among the few preventive measures that we have available to combat this pandemic, frequent and adequate handwashing seems to be an effective approach that a substantial number of college students are not practicing. Hence, this study provides direction for designing efficacious, brief educational interventions to promote handwashing. The scale utilized was psychometrically robust and met the acceptable criteria for validity and reliability and can be used for future cross-sectional and interventional studies.

However, this study has some limitations, which merit discussion. First, this study is based on only one large, public Southern U.S. university. Therefore, the findings may not be extrapolated to students of other institutions, and caution should be applied while interpreting the results. However, our sample was nearly representative of the institution where study took place. University racial breakdown for previous year was White/Caucasian (73.7%), Black/African American (4.4%), Hispanic (8.6%), and Asian (2.5%) (available at https://oir.uark.edu/quickfacts/factbook-2019-2020.pdf.

Second, the study relied on self-reported information, which can subject to measurement error. However, when it comes to measuring attitudes towards health behavior, this is the only method for the measurement. Third, in testing the instrument's reliability, the instrument's stability over time was not assessed. This offers a potential avenue for future research and will be especially important before conducting experimental studies. Fourth, actual availability of resources for handwashing were not measured in this study. Finally, the study used a cross-sectional design in which the independent and dependent variables are measured simultaneously, thereby preventing any causal inferences.

5. Conclusions

Amid the COVID-19 pandemic, this is a timely study that identifies a newer fourth-generation behavior change theory, MTM, to address handwashing behavior among college students. This study found that a substantial number of college students are not following handwashing recommendations. Further, the study provided evidence that MTM can help promote handwashing behavior among college students. There is a need to design and test individual-level behavior change interventions and media campaigns based on MTM for efficacy and effectiveness to change handwashing behavior among college students.

Author Contributions: Conceptualization, M.S. and R.E.D.; methodology, M.S., R.E.D. and K.B.; software, K.B.; validation, M.S., R.E.D., K.B. and A.H.W.; formal analysis, K.B.; investigation, all authors; resources, M.S., R.E.D. and K.B.; data curation, K.B. and M.S.; writing—original draft preparation, M.S., K.B. and A.H.W.; writing—review and editing, all authors; visualization, K.B. and M.S.; supervision, M.S., R.E.D. and K.B.; project administration, M.S., R.E.D. and K.B. All authors have read and agreed to the published version of the manuscript.

Funding: This research received no external funding.

Institutional Review Board Statement: The study was conducted according to the guidelines of the Declaration of Helsinki and approved by the Institutional Review Board (or Ethics Committee) of University of Arkansas (protocol ID: 2009281493 approved on 09/21/2020).

Informed Consent Statement: Informed consent was obtained from all subjects involved in the study.

Data Availability Statement: The data presented in this study are available on request from the corresponding author. The data are not publicly available due to ethical reasons.

Conflicts of Interest: The authors declare no conflict of interest.

References

1. Bruinen de Bruin, Y.; Lequarre, A.S.; McCourt, J.; Peter, C.; Filippo, P.; Maryam, Z.; Jeddid, C.; Colosioe, M.G. Initial impacts of global risk mitigation measures taken during the combatting of the COVID-19 pandemic. *Saf. Sci.* **2020**, *128*, 104773. [CrossRef]
2. World Health Organization. Coronavirus Disease (COVID-19) Pandemic. 2020. Available online: https://www.who.int/emergencies/diseases/novel-coronavirus-2019 (accessed on 11 November 2020).
3. Centers for Disease Control and Prevention. United States COVID-19 Cases and Deaths by State. 2020. Available online: https://covid.cdc.gov/covid-data-tracker/#cases_casesper100klast7days (accessed on 18 November 2020).
4. Centers for Disease Control and Prevention. How to Protect Yourself & Others. 2020. Available online: https://www.cdc.gov/coronavirus/2019-ncov/prevent-getting-sick/prevention.html (accessed on 18 November 2020).
5. World Health Organization. Coronavirus Disease (COVID-19) Advice for the Public. 2020. Available online: https://www.who.int/emergencies/diseases/novel-coronavirus-2019/advice-for-public (accessed on 11 November 2020).
6. Aiello, A.E.; Coulborn, R.M.; Perez, V.; Larson, E.L. Effect of hand hygiene on infectious disease risk in the community setting: A meta-analysis. *Am. J. Public Health* **2008**, *98*, 137. [CrossRef] [PubMed]
7. Freeman, M.C.; Stocks, M.E.; Cumming, O.; Aurelie, J.; Julian, P.T.H.; Jennyfer, W.; Annette, P.-U.; Sophie, B.; Paul, R.H.; Lorna, F.; et al. Hygiene and health: Systematic review of handwashing practices worldwide and update of health effects. *Trop. Med. Int. Health* **2014**, *19*, 906–916. [CrossRef]
8. Centers for Diesase Control and Prevention. Considerations for Institutions of Higher Education. 2020. Available online: https://www.cdc.gov/coronavirus/2019-ncov/community/colleges-universities/considerations.html#PlanPrepare (accessed on 11 November 2020).
9. Boehmer, T.K.; DeVies, J.; Caruso, E.; van Santen, K.L.; Shichao, T.; Carla, L.B.; Kathleen, P.H.; Aaron, K.-P.; Stephanie, D.; Matthew, L.; et al. Changing Age Distribution of the COVID-19 Pandemic—United States. *MMWR Morb. Mortal. Wkly. Rep.* **2020**, *69*, 1404–1409. [CrossRef]
10. Walke, H.T.; Honein, M.A.; Redfield, R.R. Preventing and Responding to COVID-19 on College Campuses [published online ahead of print, 29 September 2020]. *JAMA* **2020**. [CrossRef] [PubMed]
11. American College Health Association. Considerations for Reopening Institutions of Higher Education in the COVID-19 Era. 2020. Available online: https://www.acha.org/documents/resources/guidelines/ACHA_Considerations_for_Reopening_IHEs_in_the_COVID-19_Era_May2020.pdf (accessed on 11 November 2020).
12. Borchgrevink, C.P.; Cha, J.; Kim, S. Hand washing practices in a college town environment. *J. Environ. Health* **2013**, *75*, 18–24. [PubMed]
13. Drankiewicz, D.; Dundes, L. Handwashing among female college students. *Am. J. Infect. Control.* **2003**, *31*, 67–71. [CrossRef] [PubMed]
14. Resende, K.K.M.; Neves, L.F.; de Rezende, C.N.L.; Martins, L.J.O.; Costa, C.R.R. Educator and Student Hand Hygiene Adherence in Dental Schools: A Systematic Review and Meta-Analysis. *J. Dent. Educ.* **2019**, *83*, 575–584. [CrossRef]
15. Lhakhang, P.; Lippke, S.; Knoll, N.; Schwarzer, R. Evaluating brief motivational and self-regulatory hand hygiene interventions: A cross-over longitudinal design. *BMC Public Health* **2015**, *15*, 79. [CrossRef]
16. Mackert, M.; Liang, M.C.; Champlin, S. "Think the sink": Preliminary evaluation of a handwashing promotion campaign. *Am. J. Infect. Control* **2013**, *41*, 275–277. [CrossRef]
17. Zhou, G.; Jiang, T.; Knoll, N.; Schwarzer, R. Improving hand hygiene behaviour among adolescents by a planning intervention. *Psychol. Health Med.* **2015**, *20*, 824–831. [CrossRef] [PubMed]
18. Guzek, D.; Skolmowska, D.; Głąbska, D. Analysis of Gender-Dependent Personal Protective Behaviors in a National Sample: Polish Adolescents' COVID-19 Experience (PLACE-19) Study. *Int. J. Environ. Res. Public Health* **2020**, *17*, 5770. [CrossRef] [PubMed]
19. Zhang, M.; Li, Q.; Du, X.; Zip, D.; Ding, Y.; Tan, X.; Liu, Q. Health Behavior Toward COVID-19: The Role of Demographic Factors, Knowledge, and Attitude Among Chinese College Students During the Quarantine Period. *Asia Pac. J. Public Health* **2020**, 1010539520951408. [CrossRef] [PubMed]
20. Tong, K.K.; Chen, J.H.; Yu, E.W.Y.; Wu, A.M. Adherence to COVID-19 Precautionary Measures: Applying the Health Belief Model and Generalized Social Beliefs to a Probability Community Sample. *Appl. Psychol. Health Well Being* **2020**. [CrossRef] [PubMed]
21. Sharma, M. Multi-theory model (MTM) for health behavior change. *Webmed. Cent. Behav.* **2015**, *6*, WMC004982.
22. Knowlden, A.P.; Sharma, M.; Nahar, V.K. Using multitheory model of health behavior change to predict adequate sleep behavior. *Fam. Community Health* **2017**, *40*, 56–61. [CrossRef]
23. Nahar, V.K.; Wilkerson, A.H.; Stephens, P.M.; Kim, R.W.; Sharma, M. Using the multitheory model to predict initiation and sustenance of physical activity behavior among osteopathic medical students. *J. Am. Osteopath Assoc.* **2019**, *119*, 479–487. [CrossRef]
24. Sharma, M.; Catalano, H.P.; Nahar, V.K.; Lingam, V.; Johnson, P.; Ford, M.A. Using multi-theory model of health behavior change to predict portion size consumption among college students. *Health Promot. Perspect.* **2016**, *6*, 137–144. [CrossRef]

25. Sharma, M.; Anyimukwu, C.; Kim, R.W.; Nahar, V.K.; Ford, M.A. Predictors of responsible drinking or abstinence among college students who binge drink: A multitheory model approach. *J. Am. Osteopath. Assoc.* **2018**, *118*, 519–530. [CrossRef]
26. Sharma, M.; Stephens, P.M.; Nahar, V.K.; Catalano, H.P.; Lingam, V.; Ford, M.A. Using multi-theory model to predict initiation and sustenance of fruit and vegetable consumption among college students. *J. Am. Osteopath Assoc.* **2018**, *118*, 507–517. [CrossRef]
27. Sharma, M.; Largo-Wight, E.; Kanekar, A.; Kusumoto, H.; Hooper, S.; Nahar, V.K. Using the multi-theory model (MTM) of health behavior change to explain intentional outdoor nature contact behavior among college students. *Int. J. Environ. Res. Public Health* **2020**, *17*, 6104. [CrossRef]
28. Ajzen, I. The theory of planned behavior. *Organ. Behav. Hum. Decis. Process* **1991**, *50*, 179–211. [CrossRef]
29. Bandura, A. Health promotion by social cognitive means. *Health Educ. Behav.* **2004**, *31*, 143–164. [CrossRef] [PubMed]
30. Freire, P. *Pedagogy of the Oppressed*; Continuum International Publishing Group Inc.: New York, NY, USA, 1970.
31. Goleman, D. *Emotional Intelligence*; Bantam: New York, NY, USA, 1995.
32. Misro, A.; Hussain, M.; Jones, T.; Baxter, M.; Khanduja, V. A quick guide to survey research. *Ann. R Coll. Surg. Engl.* **2014**, *96*, 87–89. [CrossRef] [PubMed]
33. Eysenbach, G. Correction: Improving the quality of web surveys: The checklist for reporting results of internet E-surveys (Cherries). *J. Med. Int. Res.* **2012**, *14*, e8. [CrossRef]
34. Centers for Disease Control and Prevention. When and How to Wash Your Hands. 2020. Available online: https://www.cdc.gov/handwashing/when-how-handwashing.html (accessed on 11 November 2020).
35. Sharma, M. *Theoretical Foundations of Health Education and Health Promotion*, 3rd ed.; Jones and Bartlett: Burlington, MA, USA, 2017; pp. 250–262.
36. Sharma, M.; Petosa, R.L. *Measurement and Evaluation for Health Educators*, 1st ed.; Jones & Bartlett Learning: Burlington, MA, USA, 2014.
37. Kaiser, H.F. The application of electronic computers to factor Analysis. *Educ. Psychol. Meas.* **1960**, *20*, 141–151. [CrossRef]
38. Stevens, J. *Applied Multivariate Statistics for the Social Sciences*, 3rd ed.; Lawrence Erlbaum Associates: Mahwah, NJ, USA, 1996.
39. Faul, F.; Erdfelder, E.; Buchner, A.; Lang, A.G. Statistical power analyses using G*Power 3.1: Tests for correlation and regression analyses. *Behav. Res. Methods* **2009**, *41*, 1149–1160. [CrossRef]
40. Arbianingsih, U.Y.; Rustina, Y.; Krianto, T.; Ayubi, D. Arbi Care application increases preschool children's hand-washing self-efficacy among preschool children. *Enferm. Clin.* **2018**, *28* (Suppl. 1), 27–30. [CrossRef]
41. Contzen, N.; Inauen, J. Social-cognitive factors mediating intervention effects on handwashing: A longitudinal study. *J. Behav. Med.* **2015**, *38*, 956–969. [CrossRef]
42. Karadag, E. The effect of a self-management program on handwashing/mask-wearing behaviours and self-efficacy level in peritoneal dialysis patients: A pilot study. *J. Ren. Care* **2019**, *45*, 93–101. [CrossRef]
43. Rosen, L.; Zucker, D.; Brody, D.; Engelhard, D.; Manor, O. The effect of a handwashing intervention on preschool educator beliefs, attitudes, knowledge and self-efficacy. *Health Educ. Res.* **2009**, *24*, 686–698. [CrossRef] [PubMed]
44. Nahar, V.K.; Sharma, M.; Catalano, H.P.; Ickes, M.J.; Johnson, P.; Ford, M.A. Testing multi-theory model (MTM) in predicting initiation and sustenance of physical activity behavior among college students. *Health Promot. Perspect.* **2016**, *6*, 58–65. [CrossRef] [PubMed]
45. Sharma, M.; Catalano, H.P.; Nahar, V.K.; Lingam, V.; Johnson, P.; Ford, M.A. Using multi-theory model (MTM) of health behavior change to predict water consumption instead of sugar sweetened beverages. *J. Res. Health Sci.* **2017**, *17*, e00370. [PubMed]
46. Gross, J.J. Emotion regulation: Affective, cognitive, and social consequences. *Psychophysiology* **2020**, *39*, 281–291. [CrossRef]
47. Hiral, M.; Graham, J.P.; Mattson, K.D.; Kelsey, A.; Mukherji, S.; Cronin, A.A. Exploring determinants of handwashing with soap in Indonesia: A quantitative analysis. *Int. J. Environ. Res. Public Health* **2016**, *13*, 868.
48. Mbakaya, B.C.; Kalembo, F.W.; Zgambo, M. Use, adoption, and effectiveness of tippy-tap handwashing station in promoting hand hygiene practices in resource-limited settings: A systematic review. *BMC Public Health* **2020**, *20*, 1005. [CrossRef]
49. Travasso, C. Emotional motivators help to increase handwashing with soap, Indian study finds. *BMJ* **2014**, *348*, g2170. [CrossRef]
50. Willmott, M.; Nicholson, A.; Busse, H.; MacArthur, G.J.; Brookes, S.; Campbell, R. Effectiveness of hand hygiene interventions in reducing illness absence among children in educational settings: A systematic review and meta-analysis. *Arch. Dis. Child.* **2016**, *101*, 42–50. [CrossRef]
51. Bashirian, S.; Barati, M.; Sharma, M.; Abasi, H.; Karami, M. Water pipe smoking reduction in the male adolescent students: An educational intervention using multi-theory model. *J. Res. Health Sci.* **2019**, *19*, e00438.
52. Brown, L.; Sharma, M.; Leggett, S.; Sung, J.H.; Bennett, R.L.; Azevedo, M. Efficacy testing of the SAVOR (Sisters Adding Fruits and Vegetables for Optimal Results) intervention among African American women: A randomized controlled trial. *Health Promot. Perspect.* **2020**, *10*, 270–280. [CrossRef]
53. Hayes, T.; Sharma, M.; Shahbazi, M.; Sung, J.H.; Bennett, R.; Reese-Smith, J. The evaluation of a fourth-generation multi-theory model (MTM) based intervention to initiate and sustain physical activity in African American women. *Health Promot. Perspect.* **2019**, *9*, 13–23. [CrossRef] [PubMed]

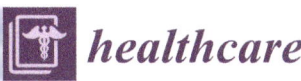

Article

Face Mask Usage among Young Polish People during the COVID-19 Epidemic—An Evolving Scenario

Radomir Reszke [1], Marta Szepietowska [2], Piotr K. Krajewski [1] Łukasz Matusiak [1], Rafał Białynicki-Birula [1] and Jacek C. Szepietowski [1,*]

[1] Department of Dermatology, Venereology and Allergology, Wrocław Medical University, 50-368 Wrocław, Poland; radomir.reszke@umed.wroc.pl (R.R.); piokrzykrajewski@gmail.com (P.K.K.); luke71@interia.pl (Ł.M.); rafal.bialynicki-birula@umed.wroc.pl (R.B.-B.)

[2] Students' Research Group of Experimental Dermatology, Department of Dermatology, Venereology and Allergology, Wrocław Medical University, 50-368 Wrocław, Poland; marta.szepietowska@student.umed.wroc.pl

* Correspondence: jacek.szepietowski@umed.wroc.pl; Tel.: +48-71-784-22-86

Abstract: The usage of face masks has been mandated in many countries in an attempt to diminish the spread of SARS-CoV-2. In this cross-sectional study, we aimed to determine face mask-wearing behaviors and practices in 1173 young Polish people during the second wave of the COVID-19 epidemic in October 2020. The majority of respondents (97.4%) declared that they wore face masks in areas/situations where it is mandatory. The most common types of utilized face masks were cloth masks (47.7%) and surgical masks (47%), followed by respirators (N95/FFP3) (3.2%) and half-face elastomeric respirators (0.9%). Over 38% reported frequently disinfecting their face masks, especially females. Respondents reporting personal atopic predisposition (64.5% vs. 72.1%; $p = 0.02$) or sensitive skin (65.5% vs. 74.3%; $p = 0.005$) declared multiple use of face masks less commonly than other individuals. Individuals suffering from facial skin lesions declared disinfecting face masks more commonly (40.8% vs. 34.9%; $p = 0.04$). Overall, the self-declared utilization of face masks among young people in Poland has improved since the beginning of the epidemic as compared with our previous study. Until the mass vaccination of the public is achieved and government policy is changed, face mask use remains a valuable tool to decrease the transmission of SARS-CoV-2.

Keywords: face masks; COVID-19; young people; behaviors

1. Introduction

Since the beginning of the COVID-19 pandemic, all countries have been subjected to a situation largely unknown previously. Over a year since pandemic onset (as of 26 April 2021), the number of confirmed cases of SARS-CoV-2 infection exceeds 146.8 million worldwide, with over 3.1 million confirmed deaths [1]. Concurrently, the epidemic situation remained concerning throughout the entire European Union. For example, the total number of confirmed COVID-19 cases in Poland has exceeded 2.7 million (26 April 2021), claiming at least 65,000 officially reported deaths [2]. Owing to the dominance of airborne transmission of SARS-CoV-2 between humans [3] and unavailability of a specific vaccine, prophylactic safety precautions instigated by each individual, endorsed and verified by relevant official services, constituted the crucial step to decrease the development of the pandemic in 2020. The World Health Organization (WHO) and European Centre for Disease Prevention and Control (ECDC) recommendations were aimed at the general public and focused on social distancing, hand hygiene, and usage of personal protective equipment (PPE) [4,5]. These recommendations were also reflected in the official regulations issued by the Polish Government [6,7], which forbade certain activities (e.g., social gatherings, running hotel or restaurant businesses), while particular behaviors became mandatory. An example of the latter is the obligation to strictly cover the nose and the mouth either with face masks or alternatively with a piece of clothing in certain places and routine everyday situations. These include workplaces, public transport, streets, shops, or churches. There is some evidence that the use of face masks may contribute to the prevention of SARS-CoV-2 spread [8,9]. According to Leffler et al. [10], in countries with cultural norms or official regulations which supported face mask-wearing, the COVID-19 epidemic resulted in an average per-capita mortality increase by 16.2% each week. In contrast, other countries experienced a 61.9% weekly mortality increase. More frequent usage of face masks during the COVID-19 pandemic is associated not only with better physical, but also mental health in terms of anxiety, depression, and stress, as recounted in a study comparing Chinese and Polish respondents [11].

Despite the literature evidence and official regulations, these factors still cannot guarantee that each person will continue to wear face masks during the pandemic. Unsurprisingly, there have been significant differences in mask-wearing behaviors and practices during the COVID-19 pandemic in the general public [12–15]. It seems that certain factors, such as age, sex, education, or dwelling location might affect the face mask-wearing prevalence and/or type of mask used. The possible associations between age and face mask-wearing behaviors are particularly interesting. Firstly, certain studies reported that younger age is related to diminished compliance with face mask-wearing recommendations [13,14,16]. There are multiple causes of this observation, such as certain common inconveniences (e.g., breathing difficulties, sweating, misting of the glasses) [17] which can occur regardless of age. Unfortunately, some individuals regard obligatory face mask usage as a restriction of personal freedom and unethical [18,19]. Secondly, younger people infected with SARS-CoV-2 are relatively more prone to experience an asymptomatic course of COVID-19 [20,21]. Consequently, they do not actively seek medical advice and continue with their usual everyday activities. Additionally, the phenomenon of superspreading deserves particular attention as well. A superspreading event (SSE) refers to a situation in which particular individuals can infect an unusually high number of secondary cases, as reviewed by Lloyd-Smith et al. [22]. The SSE seems to play an important role in the transmission of SARS-CoV-2 [23–25]. In a study based on contact tracing, it was revealed that 19% of all detected cases were in fact responsible for 80% of the entire local transmission of SARS-CoV-2 [23]. Epidemiological data from the USA support that SARS-CoV-2 superspreading might also be associated with age. The group of non-elderly (<60 years) subjects with COVID-19 was 2.78 times more likely to spread the infection than the elderly [24], whereas at least 65 out of 100 SARS-CoV-2 infections originated from people aged 20–49 [25]. Such tendencies among age groups may be explained by different associated factors, e.g., occupation or lifestyle.

Notably, due to the prolonged and evolving nature of the COVID-19 pandemic, different epidemiological regulations and restrictions were issued by the authorities. As they changed over time, this could have stimulated confusion and impeded compliance [26]. The dynamic course of the epidemic situation could have also contributed to a scenario in which certain attitudes and behaviors of the general public regarding the use of PPE have also changed over time. Therefore, our study aimed to evaluate the prevalence and detailed characteristics of face mask-wearing behaviors and practices, focusing on young Polish people during the second wave of COVID-19, seven months after the first confirmed case in Poland.

2. Materials & Methods

Our study was conducted using an original online survey developed in Google Forms® and subsequently sent to young Polish people, mainly students. Participation in the study was voluntary, with WhatsApp®, Facebook®, e-mail, or SMS invitation containing a direct link to the questionnaire. Based on the snowball sampling technique [27], each participant was able to send the link further and invite additional participants. We have gathered demographic data, as well as detailed characteristics of self-reported face mask-wearing behaviors and practices, including the type of face masks used, disinfection practices, multiple uses of face masks, as well as the personal history of atopic predisposition, sensitive skin, and facial skin lesions. We intended to perform statistical analysis with a particular emphasis on sex and the presence of skin-related conditions, as previous studies revealed their associations with face mask-wearing practices and behaviors [13,17,28,29]. Data collection occurred between 1–7 October 2020, during the second wave of the COVID-19 epidemic in Poland. The chosen time period was intentional, as it directly preceded the portended reintroduction of official government restrictions and regulations on 9 October 2020 [7]. Prior to those, it had been necessary to wear face masks in closed spaces (e.g., shops), whereas in open spaces (e.g., streets) it had been voluntary, although recommended. Since the introduction of the regulations on October 9th, strict face covering was mandated, either with a face mask or cloth, in various locations and situations in public space. These included public transport, streets, squares, cemeteries, promenades, boulevards, parking lots, and a variety of buildings (offices, schools, banks, shops, healthcare facilities, churches). In total, 1173 individuals aged 20.9 ± 2.9 years (mean $\pm$ standard deviation [SD]; range 17–27 years) provided data for further analysis. The number of included participants provided a confidence level of 95%, with a 2.86% margin of error. The majority of respondents in our cohort were females (74.7% vs. 25.3%). Statistical analysis was performed with Statistica 13 software (Dell, Inc, Round Rock, TX, USA) using the Chi-square test. A p-value less than 0.05 was considered as statistically significant. The study was performed based on the statutory activity of the department, in accordance with the ethical approval of the Wrocław Medical University Institutional Review Board (ST.C260.18.019).

3. Results

3.1. Basic Results

The vast majority of our cohort (97.4%) declared that they "often" or "always" wear face masks in areas/situations where it was mandatory. This tendency was also more frequent among females (98.3% vs. 95%; $p = 0.002$). On the other hand, 23% declared that they wear face masks "often" or "always" in areas or situations where it is not mandatory. The most common types of used face masks were cloth (47.7%) and surgical masks (47%), followed by respirators (N95/FFP3) (3.2%) and half-face elastomeric respirators (0.9%) (Table 1). Multiple-use face masks were used by 24.9% of subjects, while 69.6% declared that they use their face masks multiple times (regardless of whether the mask is designed to do so or not). Over one-third (38.3%) reported that they regularly disinfected their face masks, especially females (40.1% vs. 33%; $p = 0.03$). Regarding skin-related conditions reported by our cohort, personal atopic predisposition concerned 33.8%, with a similar prevalence in both sexes. Furthermore, sensitive skin (52.3%) and current presence of facial skin lesions (57.5%) were both reported more commonly by females (60.7% vs. 26.9%; $p < 0.0001$; and 62.6% vs. 42.4%; $p < 0.0001$; respectively).

Table 1. The basic results of the entire cohort according to sex. The *p*-values in bold were considered statistically significant.

Characteristics	Entire Cohort	Females	Males	*p*-Value
N (%)	1173	876 (74.7%)	297 (25.3%)	-
Age (mean ± SD) (years)	20.9 ± 2.9	20.9 ± 2.0	21.2 ± 4.5	$p = 0.65$
Type of face mask used				
Cloth	560 (47.7%)	426 (48.6%)	134 (45.1%)	$p = 0.29$
Surgical	552 (47.0%)	409 (46.7%)	143 (48.1%)	$p = 0.66$
Respirator (N95/FFP3)	37 (3.2%)	25 (2.9%)	12 (4.0%)	$p = 0.31$
Half-face elastomeric respirator	10 (0.9%)	6 (0.7%)	4 (1.4%)	$p = 0.28$

Table 1. *Cont.*

Characteristics	Entire Cohort	Females	Males	p-Value
None	14 (1.2%)	10 (1.1%)	4 (1.4%)	p = 0.79
Only multiple-use face masks	292 (24.9%)	225 (25.7%)	67 (22.6%)	p = 0.28
Behaviors associated with face mask use				
Face masks worn in areas/situations where it is mandatory ("often" or "always")	1143 (97.4%)	861 (98.3%)	282 (95.0%)	**p = 0.002**
Face masks worn in areas/situations where it is not mandatory ("often" or "always")	270 (23.0%)	192 (21.9%)	78 (26.3%)	p = 0.12
Disinfection	449 (38.3%)	351 (40.1%)	98 (33.0%)	**p = 0.03**
Multiple use of face masks	613 (69.6%)	445 (68.4%)	168 (73.0%)	p = 0.18
Skin-related conditions				
Personal atopic predisposition	396 (33.8%)	309 (35.3%)	87 (29.3%)	p = 0.06
Sensitive skin	613 (52.3%)	532 (60.7%)	81 (26.9%)	**p < 0.0001**
Current facial skin lesions	674 (57.5%)	548 (62.6%)	126 (42.4%)	**p < 0.0001**

3.2. Skin-Related Conditions and Their Influence on the Type of Face Masks Used and Face Mask-Related Behaviours

Individuals with personal atopic predisposition were less likely than their healthy peers to use face masks multiple times (64.5% vs. 72.1%; $p = 0.02$) (Table 2). Similarly, multiple uses of face masks were also less common among those with sensitive skin (65.5% vs. 74.3%; $p = 0.005$) (Table 3). Additionally, individuals who reported the current presence of facial skin lesions were more prone to disinfect face masks than those with healthy skin (40.8% vs. 34.9%; $p = 0.04$) (Table 4). The presence or absence of skin-related conditions did not favor our participants' habit of wearing masks in areas/situations in which their use was mandatory or not. Personal atopic predisposition ($p = 0.26$), sensitive skin ($p = 0.98$) and facial skin lesions ($p = 0.58$) did not seem to influence the participants' choice of particular type of face mask.

Table 2. The influence of personal atopic predisposition on the type of face mask used and other face mask-related behaviors. The values in bold are considered statistically significant.

Characteristics	Atopic Predisposition (n = 396)	No Atopic Predisposition (n = 777)	p-Value
Type of face mask used			
Cloth	183 (46.2%)	377 (48.5%)	p = 0.45
Surgical	186 (47.0%)	366 (47.1%)	p = 0.97
Respirator (N95/FFP3)	18 (4.5%)	19 (2.4%)	p = 0.05
Half-face elastomeric respirator	5 (1.3%)	5 (0.7%)	p = 0.28
None	4 (1.0%)	10 (1.3%)	p = 0.68
Only multiple-use face masks	100 (25.3%)	192 (24.7%)	p = 0.84

Table 2. Cont.

Characteristics	Atopic Predisposition (n = 396)	No Atopic Predisposition (n = 777)	p-Value
Behaviors associated with face mask use			
Face masks worn in areas/situations where it is mandatory ("often" or "always")	387 (97.7%)	756 (97.3%)	p = 0.66
Face masks worn in areas/situations where it is not mandatory ("often" or "always")	90 (23.7%)	180 (23.2%)	p = 0.87
Disinfection	165 (41.7%)	284 (36.6%)	p = 0.09
Multiple use of face masks	191 (64.5%)	422 (72.1%)	**p = 0.02**

Table 3. The influence of sensitive skin on the type of face mask used and other face mask-related behaviors. The values in bold are considered statistically significant.

Characteristics	Sensitive Skin (n = 613)	No Sensitive Skin (n = 560)	p-Value
Type of face mask used			
Cloth	292 (47.6%)	268 (47.9%)	p = 0.94
Surgical	287 (46.8%)	265 (47.3%)	p = 0.86
Respirator (N95/FFP3)	20 (3.3%)	17 (3.0%)	p = 0.82
Half-face elastomeric respirator	6 (1.0%)	4 (0.7%)	p = 0.62
None	8 (1.3%)	6 (1.1%)	p = 0.71
Only multiple-use face masks	140 (22.8%)	152 (27.1%)	p = 0.09
Behaviors associated with face mask use			
Face masks worn in areas/situations where it is mandatory ("often" or "always")	597 (97.4%)	546 (97.5%)	p = 0.91
Face masks worn in areas/situations where it is not mandatory ("often" or "always")	155 (25.3%)	115 (20.5%)	p = 0.05
Disinfection	248 (40.5%)	201 (35.9%)	p = 0.11
Multiple use of face masks	310 (65.5%)	303 (74.3%)	**p = 0.005**

Table 4. The influence of facial skin lesions on the type of face mask used and other face mask-related behaviors. The values in bold are considered statistically significant.

Characteristics	Facial Skin Lesions (n = 674)	No Facial Skin Lesions (n = 499)	p-Value
Type of face mask used			
Cloth	326 (48.4%)	234 (46.9%)	p = 0.62
Surgical	319 (47.3%)	233 (46.7%)	p = 0.83
Respirator (N95/FFP3)	18 (2.7%)	19 (3.8%)	p = 0.27
Half-face elastomeric respirator	4 (0.6%)	6 (1.2%)	p = 0.26
None	7 (1.0%)	7 (1.4%)	p = 0.57
Only multiple-use face masks	173 (25.7%)	119 (23.9%)	p = 0.48

Table 4. Cont.

Characteristics	Facial Skin Lesions (n = 674)	No Facial Skin Lesions (n = 499)	p-Value
Behaviors associated with face mask use			
Face masks worn in areas/situations where it is mandatory ("often" or "always")	660 (97.9%)	483 (96.8%)	p = 0.23
Face masks worn in areas/situations where it is not mandatory ("often" or "always")	162 (24.0%)	108 (21.6%)	p = 0.34
Disinfection	275 (40.8%)	174 (34.9%)	p = 0.04
Multiple use of face masks	348 (69.5%)	265 (69.7%)	p = 0.93

4. Discussion

It seems reasonable to expect that in countries with a cultural habit of wearing face masks (e.g., Japan) [30], this behavior would be easier to achieve during the ongoing COVID-19 pandemic. Conversely, and despite the epidemic situation, it cannot be ensured that the general public in other countries would adhere to the official mandatory regulations, even when the lack of compliance may result in penalties such as being fined by police or sanitary inspectors. The discussion on personal safety behaviors of the general population may focus on different baseline aspects, with age being one of the most important. Luo et al. [31] postulated that there is a generational gap in terms of undertaking preventive measures recommended by the CDC against SARS-CoV-2, with elderly individuals being more prone to abide by them. There are multiple possible explanations, ranging from higher risk of hospitalization, severe course, and fatal outcome of COVID-19 in the elderly [13,32] to more common adherence to the social norms in their area of residence [33]. Unsurprisingly, some publications revealed that wearing face masks during the COVID-19 pandemic is insufficient among young adults [13,16,28,33–35]. As an example, an American study by Haischer et al. [13] reported that among 5517 individuals entering shops in the state of Wisconsin, only 41.5% wore masks. When accounting for age groups, younger subjects (2–30 years old) wore face masks less commonly (37%) than middle-aged (30–65 years) (41%) or elderly (>65 years) (57%). Adjusted odds ratio (aOR) for a middle-aged wearing a face mask was 1.597 higher than for younger individuals (95% confidence interval [CI] 1.359–1.877), while the proportion was even higher when comparing elderly vs. younger individuals (aOR 3.434; 95% CI 2.811–4.195). Likewise, a study conducted on the Spanish population revealed that young individuals (aged 18–25 years) were least likely to wear face masks when compared to all the other age groups [33]. Consequently, in our previous study, we assessed the face mask usage prevalence and mask-related behaviors and practices, deciding to strictly focus attention on young Polish people [12]. The latter study was conducted during the first COVID-19 wave in Poland in April 2020, shortly before the introduction of the first official governmental policy which included mandatory face mask-wearing in public [6]. Therein, out of 2307 young individuals, only 60.4% admitted to wearing face masks, regardless of sex [12]. In contrast, the current study revealed that 97.4% of young respondents wore face masks in mandatory areas/situations during the second COVID-19 wave in October 2020. Although the cohorts were different in both studies and do not justify performing a direct comparison, there was a tendency for higher adherence to the safety regulations throughout the course of the epidemic in Poland. Strzelecki et al. [36] observed a correlation between the spread of the COVID-19 epidemic in Poland and Google Trends searches on PPE, including face masks. We deem these results as important evidence that, as the epidemic develops, people actively broaden their knowledge by seeking health- or life-preserving solutions, as the first step to more frequent and successful usage of PPE. They are also in line with the dynamics of our current and past [12] observations that a change in health-preserving behaviors is a process that occurs over time. Interestingly, the current study revealed that females were more compliant with the face mask-wearing regime (98.3% vs. 95.0%; $p = 0.002$), confirming the findings of previous studies [13,28]. In the setting of an epidemic, women have a crucial role in promoting preventive behaviors among their family members and social community [37]. Notably, 23% of participants also reported that they wear face masks in areas/situations where it is not mandatory. Such careful behavior may be beneficial in certain situations, e.g., when both healthy and COVID-19 positive households wear face masks. Thereby, as reported by Chinese investigators, SARS-CoV-2 transmission to other family members may be reduced by 79%. However, Wang et al. [9] noted that the primary cases needed to wear face masks before the onset of symptoms, whereas later introduction did not seem to play a protective role.

We determined that young people mostly used cloth face masks (47.7%), closely followed by surgical face masks (47%), while respirators (3.2%) and half-face elastomeric respirators (0.9%) were worn less commonly. Still, over half of our cohort utilized face masks with better protective properties (filtration efficacy) than cloth masks [38,39]. In our previous study [12], cloth face masks were also the most frequently used modality (46.2%), while surgical masks (39%) were employed relatively less commonly. The changes in cloth vs. surgical mask usage over time might stem from the fact that, during the initial stages of the epidemic, there was a shortage of surgical masks supply, making it necessary to rely on cloth masks, which are also easier to manufacture. On the other hand, the use of respirators in October 2020 (4.1% in total) was much lower than in April 2020 (14.1% in total). With a more serious epidemic scenario later in 2020, we would expect the general public to use gear with better protection properties, especially acknowledging its better availability over time. Nevertheless, due to their cost, respirators might be in fact less suitable for the general public to use daily. Regarding the impact of baseline skin conditions on face mask-wearing behaviors, the participants of our study with an atopic predisposition or sensitive skin were less prone to use face masks multiple times. Several recent studies have proven the association between face mask usage during the COVID-19 pandemic and diverse cutaneous problems [12,40,41], including the exacerbation of atopic dermatitis predominantly in mask-covered areas [42]. Multiple use of a single face mask could be associated with friction, warmth, and moisture. Additionally, the presence of formaldehyde and other preservatives could predispose to contact dermatitis [41]. These tendencies may be more pronounced, especially in a person with an atopic predisposition or sensitive skin. We also theorize that people with such predispositions (essentially of chronic nature) may possess higher knowledge on proper health-related behaviors and consequently follow the recommendations more thoroughly. Similarly, the current presence of facial skin lesions in our cohort was associated with the more common practice of face mask disinfection. This procedure was undertaken more frequently by females and seems in accordance with a higher prevalence of sensitive skin and current facial skin lesions. People with active inflammatory skin lesions may regard their nature as purely infectious and put more emphasis on hygiene. Conversely, the use of certain chemical disinfectants could predispose to the development of allergic contact dermatitis or contact urticaria [43] and further reinforce the appearance of facial skin lesions.

Our study has several limitations. The design resulted in the self-reported nature of the data acquired from the respondents. Therefore, it is unknown whether all the participants responded to all the questions truthfully. Moreover, a recall bias could also impact the results. Due to the chosen methodology, it is impossible to determine the true response rate. Notwithstanding the frequent declaration of face mask-wearing by the young people participating in this study, it must be noted that the general public and even healthcare workers may not comply with the guidelines on proper utilization of face masks according to the WHO guidelines [29,30]. Therefore, even a high proportion of respondents assessed in a dichotomous manner (wearing vs. not wearing a mask) may not actually benefit from their seemingly protective behavior. Furthermore, despite the rationale of this study explained in precedent paragraphs, a minor limitation might stem from the study concept itself. Essentially, there are conflicting reports in the literature, some of them undermining the basic rationale of the study. As an example, in the only randomized controlled trial assessing face mask-wearing in the community (DANMASK-19), the implementation of surgical masks did not result in a significantly decreased risk of SARS-CoV-2 acquisition [44]. According to ECDC, the effectiveness of medical face masks in preventing COVID-19 in the community is small to moderate, with the certainty of the recommendation being low to moderate [45]. Additionally, our assessment of face mask-wearing behaviors strictly within the particular age group might be debatable. Despite the quoted evidence regarding inadequacies in face mask-wearing behaviors among young people [13,16,28,33–35], Howard [15] observed that it is in fact the older individuals who are slightly less likely to wear face masks. We infer that face mask-wearing is not only associated with age, as other cultural and social aspects have to be considered as well. Obviously, due to the young age of the participants, the results of our study cannot be extrapolated to the general public; the situation in other countries, especially those outside of Europe, may also differ. Finally, it is vital to avoid superficial and literal conclusions that could potentially cause harmful accusations and stigmatization towards any fraction of society.

Future evaluations on the use of face masks in the general population should ideally include other age groups from different geographic regions, while the method of assessing face mask-wearing behaviors should more be objective, perhaps by utilization of external observers. In the light of more vaccinated individuals, it would be interesting to determine if the continuous usage of face masks in mostly vaccinated societies could still contribute to the prevention of further SARS-CoV-2 spread. However, it is hoped that with mass anti-COVID-19 vaccination, there will ultimately be no need for mandatory wearing of face masks, at least in certain situations [46]. Therefore, despite the scientific value and potential influence on public health policy, even healthcare professionals may not necessarily anticipate a vast influx of such reports in the near future. Lastly, setting aside the definite eradication of SARS-CoV-2, it is unknown whether another pathogen, possibly of animal origins [47–51], will eventually emerge to reenact the pandemic scenario in the following years or decades, with mandatory re-masking yet again.

5. Conclusions

In the light of the second COVID-19 wave in October 2020, the majority of young people in Poland declared that they regularly utilized face masks, as required by official government regulations. Almost half of the respondents utilized cloth masks, closely followed by surgical masks, whereas respirators were reported rarely. Female sex was associated with a higher reported prevalence of sensitive skin and current facial skin lesions. More than one-third of the respondents utilized face mask disinfectants. Females were more likely to perform this action; when compared to males, they were also more prone to wear face masks in areas/situations where it is mandatory. In comparison to our previous study on face mask-wearing behaviors in Poland which was performed in April 2020, it seems that half a year later young people followed the recommendations more meticulously, possibly as a consequence of a more serious epidemic situation and improved awareness of safety behaviors.

Author Contributions: Conceptualization: Ł.M., P.K.K., R.B.-B., M.S., and J.C.S.; methodology: Ł.M., R.B.-B., and J.C.S.; formal analysis R.R., Ł.M., P.K.K., and J.C.S.; investigation, Ł.M., P.K.K., M.S., R.B.-B., and J.C.S.; data curation, Ł.M., P.K.K., R.R., and J.C.S.; writing—original draft preparation: R.R., J.C.S.; writing—review and editing, R.R., Ł.M., R.B.-B., and J.C.S.; visualization, R.R., P.K.K., and M.S.; supervision, Ł.M., R.B.-B., and J.C.S.; All authors have read and agreed to the published version of the manuscript.

Funding: The study received no funding.

Institutional Review Board Statement: The study was performed based on the statutory activity of the department, in accordance with the previously obtained approval of the Institutional Review Board of Wrocław Medical University (ST.C260.18.019).

Informed Consent Statement: Informed consent was obtained from all subjects involved in the study.

Data Availability Statement: The data obtained in this study may be available from the corresponding author upon a reasonable request.

Acknowledgments: The cohort evaluated in this study has been used as a control group in Krajewski, P.K.; Matusiak, Ł.; Szepietowska, M.; Białynicki-Birula, R.; Szepietowski, J.C. Increased Prevalence of Face Mask-Induced Itch in Health Care Workers. *Biology.* **2020**, 9, 451; doi:10.3390/biology9120451. We sincerely thank Robert A. Schwartz (Rutgers New Jersey Medical School, NJ, USA) for his valuable contribution regarding the English Language editing of the manuscript.

Conflicts of Interest: The authors declare no conflict of interest.

References

1. World Health Organization. WHO Coronavirus Disease (COVID-19) Dashboard. Available online: https://covid19.who.int (accessed on 26 April 2021).
2. Polish Online Service. Coronavirus: Information and Recommendations. Current Regulations and Restrictions. Available online: https://www.gov.pl/web/koronawirus/wykaz-zarazen-koronawirusem-sars-cov-2 (accessed on 26 April 2021).
3. Zhang, R.; Li, Y.; Zhang, A.L.; Wang, Y.; Molina, M.J. Identifying airborne transmission as the dominant route for the spread of COVID-19. *Proc. Natl. Acad. Sci. USA* **2020**, *117*, 14857–14863. [CrossRef]
4. World Health Organization. Coronavirus Disease (COVID-19) Advice for the Public. Available online: https://www.who.int/emergencies/diseases/novel-coronavirus-2019/advice-for-public (accessed on 26 April 2021).
5. European Centre for Disease Prevention and Control. Guidelines for the Implementation of Non-Pharmaceutical Interventions against COVID-19. Available online: https://www.ecdc.europa.eu/en/publications-data/covid-19-guidelines-non-pharmaceutical-interventions (accessed on 26 April 2021).
6. Journal of Laws of the Republic of Poland. Regulation of the Council of Ministers. 15 April 2020. No. 673. Available online: https://dziennikustaw.gov.pl/DU/2020/673 (accessed on 26 April 2021).
7. Journal of Laws of the Republic of Poland. Regulation of the Council of Ministers. 9 October 2020. No. 1758. Available online: https://dziennikustaw.gov.pl/DU/2020/1758 (accessed on 26 April 2021).
8. Cheng, V.C.-C.; Wong, S.-C.; Chuang, V.W.-M.; So, S.Y.-C.; Chen, J.H.-K.; Sridhar, S.; To, K.K.-W.; Chan, J.F.-W.; Hung, I.F.-N.; Ho, P.-L.; et al. The role of community-wide wearing of face mask for control of coronavirus disease 2019 (COVID-19) epidemic due to SARS-CoV-2. *J. Infect.* **2020**, *81*, 107–114. [CrossRef]
9. Wang, Y.; Tian, H.; Zhang, L.; Zhang, M.; Guo, D.; Wu, W.; Zhang, X.; Kan, G.L.; Lei, J.; Huo, D.; et al. Reduction of secondary transmission of SARS-CoV-2 in households by face mask use, disinfection and social distancing: A cohort study in Beijing, China. *BMJ Glob. Health* **2020**, *5*, e002794. [CrossRef] [PubMed]
10. Leffler, C.T.; Ing, E.; Lykins, J.D.; Hogan, M.C.; McKeown, C.A.; Grzybowski, A. Association of Country-wide Coronavirus Mortality with Demographics, Testing, Lockdowns, and Public Wearing of Masks. *Am. J. Trop. Med. Hyg.* **2020**, *103*, 2400–2411. [CrossRef] [PubMed]
11. Wang, C.; Chudzicka-Czupała, A.; Grabowski, D.; Pan, R.; Adamus, K.; Wan, X.; Hetnał, M.; Tan, Y.; Olszewska-Guizzo, A.; Xu, L.; et al. The Association between Physical and Mental Health and Face Mask Use during the COVID-19 Pandemic: A Comparison of Two Countries with Different Views and Practices. *Front. Psychiatry* **2020**, *11*, 569981. [CrossRef] [PubMed]
12. Matusiak, Ł.; Szepietowska, M.; Krajewski, P.K.; Białynicki-Birula, R.; Szepietowski, J.C. The use of face masks during the COVID-19 pandemic in Poland: A survey study of 2315 young adults. *Dermatol. Ther.* **2020**, *33*, e13909. [CrossRef]
13. Haischer, M.H.; Beilfuss, R.; Hart, M.R.; Opielinski, L.; Wrucke, D.; Zirgaitis, G.; Uhrich, T.D.; Hunter, S.K. Who is wearing a mask? Gender-, age-, and location-related differences during the COVID-19 pandemic. *PLoS ONE* **2020**, *15*, e0240785. [CrossRef]
14. Zhang, L.; Zhu, S.; Yao, H.; Li, M.; Si, G.; Tan, X. Study on Factors of People's Wearing Masks Based on Two Online Surveys: Cross-Sectional Evidence from China. *Int. J. Environ. Res. Public Health* **2021**, *18*, 3447. [CrossRef] [PubMed]
15. Howard, M.C. The relations between age, face mask perceptions and face mask wearing. *J. Public Health* **2021**, fdab018. [CrossRef]
16. Hutchins, H.J.; Wolff, B.; Leeb, R.; Ko, J.Y.; Odom, E.; Willey, J.; Friedman, A.; Bitsko, R.H. COVID-19 Mitigation Behaviors by Age Group—United States, April–June 2020. *MMWR Morb. Mortal. Wkly. Rep.* **2020**, *69*, 1584–1590. [CrossRef]
17. Matusiak, Ł.; Szepietowska, M.; Krajewski, P.; Białynicki-Birula, R.; Szepietowski, J.C. Inconveniences due to the use of face masks during the COVID-19 pandemic: A survey study of 876 young people. *Dermatol. Ther.* **2020**, *33*, e13567. [CrossRef]
18. Royo-Bordonada, M.A.; García-López, F.J.; Cortés, F.; Zaragoza, G.A. Face masks in the general healthy population. Scientific and ethical issues. *Gac. Sanit.* 2020. [CrossRef] [PubMed]
19. Czypionka, T.; Greenhalgh, T.; Bassler, D.; Bryant, M.B. Masks and Face Coverings for the Lay Public: A Narrative Update. *Ann. Intern. Med.* **2021**, *174*, 511–520. [CrossRef]

20. Yang, R.; Gui, X.; Xiong, Y. Comparison of Clinical Characteristics of Patients with Asymptomatic vs Symptomatic Coronavirus Disease 2019 in Wuhan, China. *JAMA Netw. Open* **2020**, *3*, e2010182. [CrossRef]
21. Davies, N.G.; Klepac, P.; Liu, Y.; Prem, K.; Jit, M.; CMMID COVID-19 Working Group; Eggo, R.M. Age-dependent effects in the transmission and control of COVID-19 epidemics. *Nat. Med.* **2020**, *26*, 1205–1211. [CrossRef]
22. Lloyd-Smith, J.O.; Schreiber, S.J.; Kopp, P.E.; Getz, W.M. Superspreading and the effect of individual variation on disease emergence. *Nature* **2005**, *438*, 355–359. [CrossRef] [PubMed]
23. Adam, D.C.; Wu, P.; Wong, J.Y.; Lau, E.H.Y.; Tsang, T.K.; Cauchemez, S.; Leung, G.M.; Cowling, B.J. Clustering and superspreading potential of SARS-CoV-2 infections in Hong Kong. *Nat. Med.* **2020**, *26*, 1714–1719. [CrossRef]
24. Lau, M.S.Y.; Grenfell, B.; Thomas, M.; Bryan, M.; Nelson, K.; Lopman, B. Characterizing superspreading events and age-specific infectiousness of SARS-CoV-2 transmission in Georgia, USA. *Proc. Natl. Acad. Sci. USA* **2020**, *117*, 22430–22435. [CrossRef] [PubMed]
25. Monod, M.; Blenkinsop, A.; Xi, X.; Hebert, D.; Bershan, S.; Tietze, S.; Baguelin, M.; Bradley, V.C.; Chen, Y.; Coupland, H. Age groups that sustain resurging COVID-19 epidemics in the United States. *Science* **2021**, *371*, eabe8372. [CrossRef]
26. Han, E.; Tan, M.M.J.; Turk, E.; Sridhar, D.; Leung, G.M.; Shibuya, K.; Asgari, N.; Oh, J.; García-Basteiro, A.L.; Hanefeld, J.; et al. Lessons learnt from easing COVID-19 restrictions: An analysis of countries and regions in Asia Pacific and Europe. *Lancet* **2020**, *396*, 1525–1534. [CrossRef]
27. Heckathorn, D.D. Snowball versus respondent-driven sampling. *Sociol. Methodol.* **2011**, *41*, 355–366. [CrossRef] [PubMed]
28. Beckage, B.; Buckley, T.E.; Beckage, M.E. Prevalence of Face Mask Wearing in Northern Vermont in Response to the COVID-19 Pandemic. *Public Health Rep.* **2021**. [CrossRef]
29. Reszke, R.; Matusiak, Ł.; Krajewski, P.K.; Szepietowska, M.; Białynicki-Birula, R.; Szepietowski, J.C. The Utilization of Protective Face Masks among Polish Healthcare Workers during COVID-19 Pandemic: Do We Pass the Exam? *Int. J. Environ. Res. Public Health* **2021**, *18*, 841. [CrossRef] [PubMed]
30. Machida, M.; Nakamura, I.; Saito, R.; Nakaya, T.; Hanibuchi, T.; Takamiya, T.; Odagiri, Y.; Fukushima, N.; Kikuchi, H.; Amagasa, S.; et al. Incorrect Use of Face Masks during the Current COVID-19 Pandemic among the General Public in Japan. *Int. J. Environ. Res. Public Health* **2020**, *17*, 6484. [CrossRef] [PubMed]
31. Luo, Y.; Cheng, Y.; Sui, M. The Moderating Effects of Perceived Severity on the Generational Gap in Preventive Behaviors during the COVID-19 Pandemic in the U.S. *Int. J. Environ. Res. Public Health* **2021**, *18*, 2011. [CrossRef]
32. Yanez, N.D.; Weiss, N.S.; Romand, J.A.; Treggiari, M.M. COVID-19 mortality risk for older men and women. *BMC Public Health* **2020**, *20*, 1742. [CrossRef]
33. Barceló, J.; Sheen, G.C. Voluntary adoption of social welfare-enhancing behavior: Mask-wearing in Spain during the COVID-19 outbreak. *PLoS ONE* **2020**, *15*, e0242764. [CrossRef]
34. Mueller, A.S.; Diefendorf, S.; Abrutyn, S.; Beardall, K.A.; Millar, K.; O'Reilly, L.; Steinberg, H.; Watkins, J.T. Youth Mask-Wearing and Social-Distancing Behavior at In-Person High School Graduations During the COVID-19 Pandemic. *J. Adolesc. Health* **2021**, *68*, 464–471. [CrossRef]
35. Davies, S.H.; Della Porta, A.; Renjilian, C.B.; Sit, L.; Ginsburg, K.R. Lessons Learned: Achieving Critical Mass in Masking Among Youth in Congregate Living. *J. Adolesc. Health* **2020**, *67*, 298–299. [CrossRef]
36. Strzelecki, A.; Azevedo, A.; Albuquerque, A. Correlation between the Spread of COVID-19 and the Interest in Personal Protective Measures in Poland and Portugal. *Healthcare* **2020**, *8*, 203. [CrossRef] [PubMed]
37. Anderson, K.M.; Stockman, J.K. Staying Home, Distancing, and Face Masks: COVID-19 Prevention among U.S. Women in The COPE Study. *Int. J. Environ. Res. Public Health* **2020**, *18*, 180. [CrossRef]
38. Santos, M.; Torres, D.; Cardoso, P.C.; Pandis, N.; Flores-Mir, C.; Medeiros, R.; Normando, A.D. Are cloth masks a substitute to medical masks in reducing transmission and contamination? A systematic review. *Braz. Oral Res.* **2020**, *34*, e123. [CrossRef]
39. Morais, F.G.; Sakano, V.K.; de Lima, L.N.; Franco, M.A.; Reis, D.C.; Zanchetta, L.M.; Jorge, F.; Landulfo, E.; Catalani, L.H.; Barbosa, H.M.J.; et al. Filtration efficiency of a large set of COVID-19 face masks commonly used in Brazil. *Aerosol. Sci. Technol.* **2021**. [CrossRef]
40. Lin, P.; Zhu, S.; Huang, Y.; Li, L.; Tao, J.; Lei, T.; Song, J.; Liu, D.; Chen, L.; Shi, Y.; et al. Adverse skin reactions among healthcare workers during the coronavirus disease 2019 outbreak: A survey in Wuhan and its surrounding regions. *Br. J. Dermatol.* **2020**, *183*, 190–192. [CrossRef] [PubMed]
41. Zuo, Y.; Hua, W.; Luo, Y.; Li, L. Skin Reactions of N95 masks and Medial Masks among Health Care Personnel: A self-report questionnaire survey in China. *Contact Dermat.* **2020**, *83*, 145–147. [CrossRef] [PubMed]
42. Damiani, G.; Gironi, L.C.; Kridin, K.; Pacifico, A.; Buja, A.; Bragazzi, N.L.; Spalkowska, M.; Pigatto, P.D.M.; Santus, P.; Young Dermatologists Italian Network; et al. Mask-induced Koebner phenomenon and its clinical phenotypes: A multicenter, real-life study focusing on 873 dermatological consultations during COVID-19 pandemics. *Dermatol. Ther.* **2021**, *34*, e14823. [CrossRef] [PubMed]
43. Di Altobrando, A.; La Placa, N.; Neri, I.; Piraccini, B.M.; Vincenzi, C. Contact dermatitis due to masks and respirators during COVID-19 pandemic: What we should know and what we should do. *Dermatol. Ther.* **2020**, *33*, e14528. [CrossRef]
44. Bundgaard, H.; Bundgaard, J.S.; Raaschou-Pedersen, D.E.T.; von Buchwald, C.; Todsen, T.; Norsk, J.B.; Pries-Heje, M.M.; Vissing, C.R.; Nielsen, P.B.; Winsløw, U.C.; et al. Effectiveness of Adding a Mask Recommendation to Other Public Health Measures to

Prevent SARS-CoV-2 Infection in Danish Mask Wearers: A Randomized Controlled Trial. *Ann. Intern. Med.* **2021**, *174*, 335–343. [CrossRef]
45. European Centre for Disease Control and Prevention. Using Face Masks in the Community: First Update—Effectiveness in Reducing Transmission of COVID-19. Available online: https://www.ecdc.europa.eu/en/publications-data/using-face-masks-community-reducing-covid-19-transmission (accessed on 26 April 2020).
46. Centers for Disease Control and Prevention. When You've Been Fully Vaccinated. How to Protect Yourself and Others. Available online: https://www.cdc.gov/coronavirus/2019-ncov/vaccines/fully-vaccinated.html (accessed on 27 April 2020).
47. Letko, M.; Seifert, S.N.; Olival, K.J.; Plowright, R.K.; Munster, V.J. Bat-borne virus diversity, spillover and emergence. *Nat. Rev. Microbiol.* **2020**, *18*, 461–471. [CrossRef]
48. Morens, D.M.; Fauci, A.S. Emerging Pandemic Diseases: How We Got to COVID-19. *Cell* **2020**, *182*, 1077–1092. [CrossRef]
49. Schwartz, R.A.; Kapila, R. Pandemics over the Centuries. *Clin. Dermatol.* **2021**, *39*, 5–8. [CrossRef] [PubMed]
50. Hashimoto, S.; Hikichi, M.; Maruoka, S.; Gon, Y. Our future: Experiencing the coronavirus disease 2019 (COVID-19) outbreak and pandemic. *Respir. Investig.* **2021**, *59*, 169–179. [CrossRef] [PubMed]
51. Halabowski, D.; Rzymski, P. Taking a lesson from the COVID-19 pandemic: Preventing the future outbreaks of viral zoonoses through a multi-faceted approach. *Sci. Total Environ.* **2021**, *757*, 143723. [CrossRef] [PubMed]

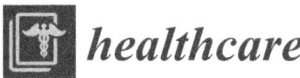 healthcare

Article

Development of a Novel Design and Subsequent Fabrication of an Automated Touchless Hand Sanitizer Dispenser to Reduce the Spread of Contagious Diseases

Arnab Das [1], Adittya Barua [1], Md. Ajwad Mohimin [1], Jainal Abedin [2], Mayeen Uddin Khandaker [3,*] and Kholoud S. Al-mugren [4]

[1] Department of Mechanical Engineering, Chittagong University of Engineering and Technology, Chittagong 4349, Bangladesh; arnabdasanik@gmail.com (A.D.); adittyabarua@yahoo.com (A.B.); ajwadmohimin@gmail.com (M.A.M.)
[2] Faculty of Public Health, Thammasat University, Bangkok 10200, Thailand; abedinj88@yahoo.com
[3] Centre for Applied Physics and Radiation Technologies, School of Engineering and Technology, Sunway University, Bandar Sunway 47500, Selangor, Malaysia
[4] Department of Physics, Princess Nourah Bint Abdulrahman University, Riyadh 11144, Saudi Arabia; ksalmogren@pnu.edu.sa
* Correspondence: mayeenk@sunway.edu.my

Abstract: Background: The use of a touchless automated hand sanitizer dispenser may play a key role to reduce contagious diseases. The key problem of the conventional ultrasonic and infra-red-based dispensers is their malfunctioning due to the interference of sunlight, vehicle sound, etc. when deployed in busy public places. To overcome such limitations, this study introduced a laser-based sensing device to dispense sanitizer in an automated touchless process. Method: The dispensing system is based on an Arduino circuit breadboard where an ATmega328p microcontroller was pre-installed. To sense the proximity, a light-dependent resistor (LDR) is used where the laser light is to be blocked after the placement of human hands, hence produced a sharp decrease in the LDR sensor value. Once the LDR sensor value exceeds the lower threshold, the pump is actuated by the microcontroller, and the sanitizer dispenses through the nozzle. Results and discussion: A novel design and subsequent fabrication of a low-cost, touchless, automated sanitizer dispenser to be used in public places, was demonstrated. The overall performance of the manufactured device was analyzed based on the cost and power consumption, and environmental factors by deploying it in busy public places as well as in indoor environment in major cities in Bangladesh, and found to be more efficient and cost-effective compared to other dispensers available in the market. A comprehensive discussion on this unique design compared to the conventional ultrasonic and infra-red based dispensers, is presented to show its suitability over the commercial ones. The guidelines of the World Health Organization are followed for the preparation of sanitizer liquid. A clear demonstration of the circuitry connections is presented herein, which facilitates the interested individual to manufacture a cost-effective dispenser device in a relatively short time and use it accordingly. **Conclusion:** This study reveals that the LDR-based automated hand sanitizer dispenser system is a novel concept, and it is cost-effective compared to the conventional ones. The presented device is expected to play a key role in contactless hand disinfection in public places, and reduce the spread of infectious diseases in society.

Keywords: novel design; fabrication; automated dispenser; LDR based controller; reduction of COVID-19 spread

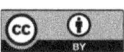

Citation: Das, A.; Barua, A.; Mohimin, M.A.; Abedin, J.; Khandaker, M.U.; Al-mugren, K.S. Development of a Novel Design and Subsequent Fabrication of an Automated Touchless Hand Sanitizer Dispenser to Reduce the Spread of Contagious Diseases. *Healthcare* **2021**, *9*, 445. https://doi.org/10.3390/healthcare9040445

Academic Editors: Manoj Sharma, Kavita Batra and Tao-Hsin Tung

Received: 8 February 2021
Accepted: 7 April 2021
Published: 10 April 2021

Publisher's Note: MDPI stays neutral with regard to jurisdictional claims in published maps and institutional affiliations.

Copyright: © 2021 by the authors. Licensee MDPI, Basel, Switzerland. This article is an open access article distributed under the terms and conditions of the Creative Commons Attribution (CC BY) license (https://creativecommons.org/licenses/by/4.0/).

1. Introduction

At present, the whole world is going through a pandemic due to coronavirus disease (COVID-19), which was first spotted in December 2019 in Wuhan, China. Since this virus is highly contagious, the World Health Organization (WHO) [1] has provided some guidelines to reduce its community transmission in various ways. One of the mandatory recommended actions is to perform hand washes/rub with soap/hand sanitizer in a frequent manner [1].

In principle, hand hygiene is now recognized as one of the most crucial issues for infection prevention and control. In the wake of the increasing severity of disease and treatment complexity, and a global pandemic superimposed by multidrug resistant (MDR) pathogen infections, the healthcare professionals (HCPs) are now returning to the basics of infection prevention by simple measures such as hand hygiene [2]. A relevant study conducted by White et al. [3] has shown a decrease of 14.8–39.9% in the upper respiratory disease symptoms among residential students (university) due to a general improvement of hand hygiene behavior.

Alcohol-based hand sanitizer (ABHS) is a useful material against the spread of infectious viruses in crowded areas such as clinics, workplaces, schools, etc. [2] It also helps to reduce the spread of disease-causing germs and bacteria. Early comprehensive research on the effectiveness of antiseptic hand rubs revealed that ABHS significantly reduces bacterial counts on hands [3]. Ehrenkranz et al. [4] reported that the ABHS is more effective in preventing the hand transfer of Gram-negative bacteria than the bland soap hand wash.

The hand sanitizer dispenser plays a significant role to allow individuals to wash/rub their hands using ABHS while on the go. A study by Fournier et al. [5] reported that the use of a strategically positioned hand sanitizer dispenser was successful in raising hand hygiene activity from 1.52% to over 60%. A few types of dispensers such as mechanical, automated with pushbuttons, touchless, etc., are available to dispense the liquid or gaseous sanitizing materials. In public places including hospitals, the use of mechanical dispensers is found widespread. Since physical contact is mandatory for using mechanical dispensers, they are vulnerable to pathogen infection. By performing a study on the hospital-based mechanical hand sanitizer dispenser, Erief et al. [6] concluded that the infected person may contaminate the dispenser which may trigger hospital-acquired infection. Automated pushbutton hand sanitizer dispensers are usually deployed in healthcare facilities, but these devices often have the possibility of being contaminated and become a center for pathogens [7]. Based on some other earlier studies [6,7], it is clear that mechanical and electrical dispensers (having a pushbutton) are vulnerable as these can be contaminated with pathogens that cause hand-associated infections (HAI). Consequently, nowadays, automated touchless sanitizers are taking place in healthcare facilities, especially in developed countries [8]. As this dispenser does not require any human contact to operate, it can be very effective to stop the spread of infectious diseases if used carefully.

A sanitizer dispenser can be made touchless automatic in different ways since various types of sensors can be used to sense the proximity [8]. Generally, ultrasound sensors [9–15] and infrared sensors [16–20] are used to make a low-cost sanitizer dispenser, but they show poor performances in public places where there is a lot of noise. Some dispensers are based on infrared radiation (IR) sensors, but they show malfunctions especially on sunny days where sunlight intensity varies because of clouds or reflection from the ground. However, such drawbacks can be easily overcome by using a light-dependent resistor (LDR) or photoresistive light sensor. In the present study, a laser light is used to block other reflections of light in the photoresistive light sensor, and this method of laser-based proximity tracking using an LDR sensor has proven to be more effective and more user friendly while considered to be used in busy public places. It is true that a large number of very low-income populations are living in the so-called developing countries like Bangladesh, Afghanistan, Cambodia, Guinea, Haiti, Laos, etc., and most of the time, some public places like bus stands, train stations, raw markets, hospitals, etc., remain crowded in those countries. The common population usually does not have the capability or is careless to maintain individual sanitization in a frequent manner. In such a situation, a touchless automated hand sanitizer dispenser is essential to stop the spreading of pathogens. Fortunately, due to the advancement of science and technology, it becomes possible to locally fabricate a low-cost automated hand sanitizer dispenser, and such a low-cost device may be very effective to be deployed in public places and individual use as well.

After a thorough analysis of both the online and offline market authors found that photo resistor sensor-based dispenser devices are not available in the market. In most of the dispenser devices, an infrared sensor is used for reducing the complexity and some devices are based on ultrasonic sensors. Based on the authors' knowledge, this unique concept of making dispenser devices using an LDR (light dependent resistor) sensor with a laser light has received less attention from the scientific community, thus forms the main subject matters of this study.

The main objective of this study is to facilitate the process of assembling and making a low-cost hand sanitizer dispenser, which is fully touchless and automated using laser detection technology. In this paper, a novel design of an automated hand sanitizer dispenser is proposed, and subsequently, fabricated using the low-cost components that are commonly available in almost every developing country. A photoelectric resistor (LDR) is used to detect human hands inside the laser detection chamber, and this sensor is perfectly compatible with both daylight and night. A comprehensive discussion of the fabricated device with respect to the conventional ones is presented to show the pros and cons of this device. Thus, this study may help to stop the COVID-19 transmission in densely populated developing countries where industrial/commercial dispensers are costly and not readily available.

2. Materials and Methods

The main objective of this study is to develop an automated hand sanitizer dispenser that will be able to reduce the spread of viruses such as COVID-19 and save people from a pandemic. The dispenser device was fabricated under two key objectives: user-friendly and cost-effective. The materials to be used in the device fabrication were selected and actuated with these goals in mind. A brief information of the hardware components together with their key features is presented in Table 1. Furthermore, an overview of the fabrication process of the dispenser device is shown via a flow chart in Figure 1.

Table 1. List of all components that were used to fabricate the automated hand sanitizer dispenser.

Major Components	Manufacturer/Brand	Advantages	Price (USD)
R3 Board ATmega328P with USB Cable for Arduino-Compatible	Kuman	• Inexpensive • Cross-platform-runs on Windows, Macintosh OSX, and Linux operating systems while other microcontroller circuits only run on windows • User-friendly programming environment	10.690
MCIGICM Photoresistor Photo Light Sensitive Resistor, Light Dependent Resistor 5 mm	MCIGICM	• Light resistance (at 10 Lux): 5–10 Kohm which is useful in this study • Perfect dark resistance: 0.5 Mohm • Good response time: 20 ms (Rise), 30 ms (Down) • Resistance illumination: 4	0.133
HiLetgo® L298N Motor Drive Controller Board Module Dual H Bridge DC Stepper For Arduino	HiLetgo®	• Over-temperature protection • Maximum supply voltage 35 V • Maximum output DC current 4 A • Low saturation voltage • Logical "0" input voltage up to 1.5 V	2.470

Table 1. Cont.

Major Components	Manufacturer/Brand	Advantages	Price (USD)
Uxcell Female DC Power Jack Socket Connector	Uxcell	• Easy to connect • Barrel connectors are not rare and used universally	1.018
HiLetgo 5V 650 nm 5 mW Red Dot Laser Head Red Laser Diode Laser Tube with Leads Head Outer Diameter 6mm	HiLetgo®	• Optimal temperature tolerance: −36~65 °C operating temperature range • Low working voltage: 5 V DC	0.599
EDGELEC 100 K ohm Resistor 1/4 w (0.25 Watt) ± 1% Tolerance Metal Film Fixed Resistor	EDGELEC	• Long working life • High temperature resistance • Moisture proof	0.057
JOVNO 12V 1A Power Supply Adapter 100–240 V AC to DC 12volt 12 W 1amp 800 mA 500 mA Power Converter Transformer with 5.5 × 2.5 mm Tip	JOVNO	• Universal adapter: • Built in automatic over-voltage protection, • Over-current protection • Over-temperature protection • Short circuit protection • Fire retardant shell	3.990
Zlolia 12 V Waterproof LED Strip Light 5 M 300LEDs	Zlolia	• Waterproof • Long life span: 50,000 h	0.010
Mini DC Brushless Water Pump JT-600C-12 16 mm Internal Thread	Zjchao	• Long life and low noise, easy to install • The pump is made of resin glue seal which is of good insulation	6.280

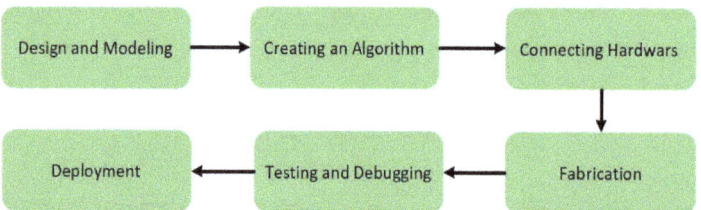

Figure 1. Flow diagram of the working process.

2.1. Design and Modeling

The performance of any device relies on different factors such as durability, the endurance of environmental change or it can be a totally psychological issue whether people are noticing the device or not. These factors mostly depend on the design or architecture of that device. The automated hand sanitizer dispenser device is designed in CAD software and the dimensions are shown in Table 2. The isometric view of the designed dispenser model is shown in Figure S1 with the dimensional parameters.

PVC flexible pipe was used in this work, which is sterile by a nontoxic, nonpyrogenic ethylene oxide (EO) gas. The pipe is divided into two sections; the diameter of the first section and the second section of the pipe is 3 and 2 mm, respectively. The first section is connected in between the motor pump and the sanitizer container, and the second section is connected to the outlet of the pump, which is directly connected to the spray nozzle/dispensing point. This nozzle is used to spray the sanitizer liquid. The two sections combined can supply 20 drops to 60 drops/mL, and it is disposable, also environmentally friendly. The rate of drops/mL is controlled by the pressure from the pump programmed into the microcontroller using Arduino IDE. The nozzle and piping system are commonly used as medical equipment for intravenous tubing for the rapid infusion of fluids. The piping system is shown in a block diagram (Figure 2a).

Table 2. Design parameters of the dispensing device.

Physical Quantity or Measurand	Parameters	Units (cm)
Basement	Length (l) × width (w)	20 × 20
Sidewall	Length, l_1, l_2	27, 32
Laser detection chamber	Height, h_c	13

l_1 = Height of the lower part of the left and right side wall of the device from the base, l_2 = Height of the upper part of the left and right wall of the device from the basement, h_c = Height of the chamber where users may put their hand palms.

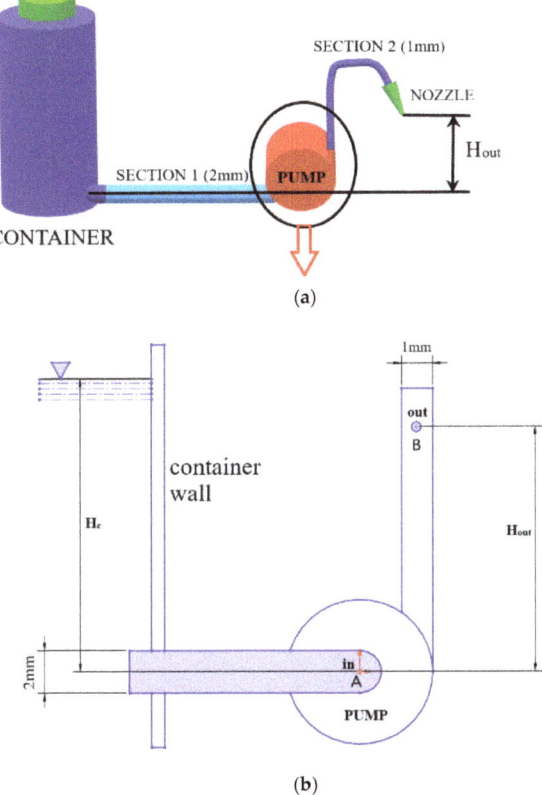

Figure 2. (a) Three-dimensional graphical representation of the piping system, (b) schematic diagram of the pump system

Theoretical Aspect

The dispenser device was designed based on some numerical assessment. The placement of the pipe in Section 1 was designed so that gravitational pull can be used to increase the fluid outlet pressure which helps to reduce the energy to be used by the motor pump to pump out the sanitizer. On the other hand, the placement of pipe in Section 2 was actuated by considering the loss of sanitizer from the nozzle due to the gravitational pressure and capillary pressure while the pump is off. This is ensured by optimizing the nozzle height based on the following calculations. The total pressure at the inlet of the pipe "Section 1" and outlet pressure at the end of the pipe "Section 2", is calculated using Bernoulli's Equations between the fluid (sanitizer) surface of the container and the fluid issuing from the nozzle [21].

$$\frac{V^2}{2g} + \frac{P}{\gamma} + Z = constant \tag{1}$$

where V is the velocity of the dispensing media, P is the pressure at specific elevation, ρ is the fluid density, g is the acceleration due to gravity, $\frac{V^2}{2g}$ is the kinetic energy, $\frac{P}{\gamma}$ is the flow work, and Z is the potential energy. Here, losses due to the minor bending of the pipe are neglected. The schematic diagram showing the parameters is shown in Figure 2b.

The amount of energy required by the pump to process per unit weight of the fluid can be calculated by Equation (2).

$$Z = \gamma Q(\Delta H) \tag{2}$$

where Q is the volumetric flow rate and ΔH is the head imparted to liquid by the pump, and γ is the specific weight which can be calculated from

$$\gamma = \rho g \tag{3}$$

where ρ is the density of the sanitizer liquid and g is the acceleration due to gravity. The velocity at pump inlet point A and outlet point B is calculated using Equations (4) and (5).

$$\text{Vin} = \frac{Q}{Area} \tag{4}$$

$$\text{Vout} = \left(\frac{r2}{r1}\right)^2 \times \text{Vin} \tag{5}$$

Then applying Bernoulli's equation to the free surface in the container and the inlet point A, taking the horizontal line through the inlet point A as the datum pressure at the pump inlet, Equation (5) gives:

$$\text{Hc} = \frac{Pin}{\gamma} + \frac{\text{Vin}^2}{2g} \tag{6}$$

Here, H_c is the distance of the centerline of the pump inlet pipe from the surface of the sanitizer inside the container. Energy per unit weight of liquid at outlet point B is greater than at A by the energy per unit weight supplied by the pump. Now applying Bernoulli's equation between A and B, the pressure at the pump outlet is calculated from Equation (6),

$$\frac{\text{Vin}^2}{2g} + \frac{Pin}{\gamma} + \Delta H = \text{Hout} + \frac{\text{Vout}^2}{2g} + \frac{Pout}{\gamma} \tag{7}$$

Here, P_{in} and P_{out} are the inlet and outlet pressures and H_{out} is the height from the pump inlet pipe axis to the nozzle. Using the similar method, the pressure and velocity at the nozzle outlet is also determined, and based on these calculations the required height of the nozzle is calculated using the constant power output value of the motor pump.

2.2. Control System and Connection

Several control systems are available in the literature such as Arduino, Raspberry pie, Teensy 3.6, Particle photon, Adafruit Feather Huzzah, Beagleboard pocket Beagle, STM32F3 Discovery. However, in this study, the control system of the dispensing device was maintained by using Arduino software. The Arduino system consists of H-bridge, Arduino board, breadboard, pushbuttons, LED, and connectors. The main reasons behind the selection of the Arduino Uno system are its low cost compared to other systems, and the suitability to be used in cross-platforms. As a result, this system is compatible with every platform—Linux operating system, windows, Macintosh OS. While other control systems are only compatible with a particular system, either Linux or Windows, or Macintosh OS. Moreover, the supported signal bandwidth and RAM also show better features in Arduino than the other aforementioned control systems. Further favorable features are that it can be operated by a USB cable or a battery with a voltage range from 7 to 20 V(Volt). To protect the board from overload, and to control the 12 V motor pump properly, an L298 motor controller system was used. Figure S2 shows the overall connections between components with the Arduino board.

2.2.1. L298 Controller Connection

This system is powered by a 12 V DC input from the adapter through a 12 V port and GND port (see in Figure 3). It has an additional 5 V port besides these two ports. A 5 V capacitive laser is connected using this 5 V port and the GND port. The system has two enable (ENA) pins along with four input pins. These pins are connected to the analog and digital pins of the Arduino board. By these pins, the microcontroller is connected to the H-bridge of the L298 driver, and thus the motor pump can be controlled.

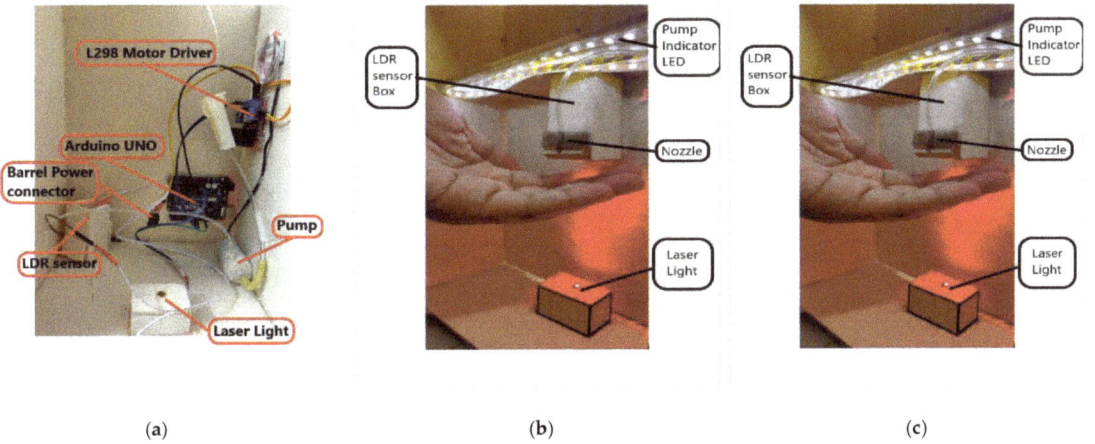

Figure 3. Original image of the proposed automated hand sanitizer dispenser; (**a**) placement of Arduino UNO, motor driver and pump, (**b**) setup of laser light, indicator LED, LDR sensor cabinet and nozzle, (**c**) sanitizer dispenser isometric view.

The motor controller has two output channels, and each channel was supplied 12 V DC. Any 12 V capacitive device can be connected using these output channels. In this study, the motor pump is connected by these channels (OUT3, OUT4). This type of connection arrangement provides an added advantage compared to conventional circuit connections. Generally, other devices operating within the range of 7–12 V can be powered directly from Arduino board (UNO). The ratings are listed below [22];

- The absolute maximum for any single IO pin is 40 mA (basically, it is the threshold at which Atmel can no longer guarantee that the chip will not be damaged);
- The total current from all the IO pins together is 200 mA max;
- The 5 V output pin is good for ~400 mA on USB, ~900 mA when using an external power adapter;
- The 900 mA is for an adapter that provides ~7 V. As the adapter voltage increases, the heat regulator has to deal with also increased values, so the maximum current will drop as the voltage increases. This is called thermal limiting.

The rating of the motor pump that is used in this study is 12 V–0.7 A; if the motor pump is directly connected to the Arduino board via GND pin and 5 V pin or other I/O pins three possible outcomes may occur:

- The pump will not run due to the low power supply;
- If the pump runs, the temperature of the voltage regulators will rise instantly and due to thermal limiting, the whole system will shut down temporarily;
- The motor pump will draw out the maximum threshold current and as a result, the chip can be damaged.

To overcome these problems L298 motor controller was used in this study which can supply DC 5 V–35 V; peak current 2 A. As a result, the motor pump can run continuously with a sufficient power supply.

2.2.2. LDR Connection

The connection of the LDR photoresistor with the Arduino board is shown in the right panel of Figure 3. Here the LDR sensor is powered from 5 V and GND pins. A 10 KΩ resistor is connected with the GND line of LDR. Arduino measures voltages from analog pins A0 to A5. On the other hand, LDR is a variable resistor whose value changes based on the intensity of light, which cannot be measured by Arduino. Therefore, to convert the varying resistance to a voltage that can be measured by Arduino directly, the LDR is used with a resistor in a potential divider circuit.

The voltage at pin A0 is measured from:

$$V_0 = \frac{5 * R1}{R1 + R2} \quad (8)$$

Here, if the resistance value of the LDR (R2) varies, the voltage at pin A0 will also vary.

2.2.3. Sanitizer Level Indicator

According to the algorithm of the present study, if the sanitizer level is lower than the threshold level, the whole process will stop. The main purpose of adding this system is to reduce power loss and also not to allow air bubbles inside the pipe through the container to pump inlet. Two probes are used here; one is connected to the 5 V pin of the Arduino circuit and the other probe is directly connected to the analog pin A1. The 5 V probe is placed at the bottom of the container and the other probe is placed just above the container outlet pipe. As a result, whenever the sanitizer level is above the limit, A1 gets a constant input signal. However, whenever below the limit, the A1-connected probe is disconnected and A1 gets "0" as a signal and the system recognizes this as the low sanitizer level.

2.3. Creating an Algorithm

An algorithm is what needed to be done before coding and fabrication. It is the step-by-step visualization of the total functionalities of the device. The working sequence of the device is depicted in a flowchart in Figure 4. A laser detection technology is used here to detect the object under the sensor and act accordingly. Whenever the LDR sensor detects a disturbance of the laser due to the hand of the user, the voltage of the photoresistor increases and the microcontroller can detect this phenomenon. Afterward, the microcontroller commands the motor driver to run the DC motor pump, which pumps out the desired amount of the sanitizing liquid from the container. Here, to ensure the desired functionality, the microcontroller is programmed according to the algorithm, considering the predictable accidental problems.

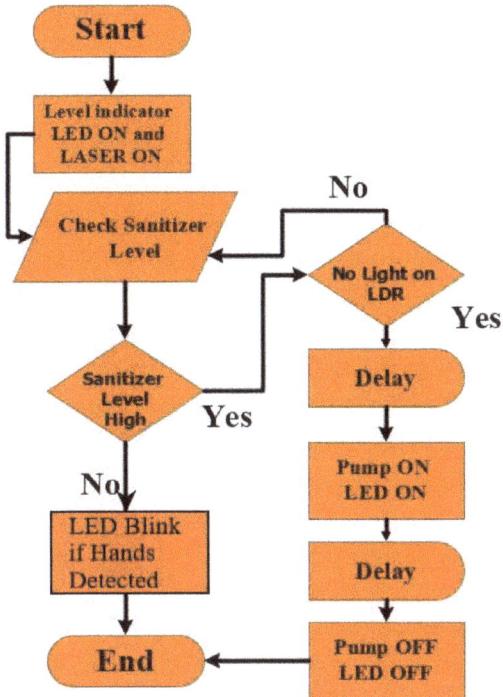

Figure 4. Flowchart of working pattern of the fabricated sanitizer dispenser.

Programming, Coding, and Debugging

Arduino IDE was used in this study to program the atmega328P microcontroller. The Arduino IDE integrated development environment offers different libraries that can be used for programming. Library functions are simple and easy to use and do not require individual microcontroller registers to be addressed in the programming. The developed coding that is used in this study is shown in Figure S3.

Here, the limit 550 declared is the threshold limit for the LDR photoresistor which is set after various trials and errors in various lighting conditions. Motor pump speed control is introduced here. The pump start speed value is set to 10 initially which will gradually increase over time by adding 2 with the previous value. After that, the pump will stop instantly to stop the sanitizer flow instantly. Here, as the pump does not speed up instantly, the durability of the pump is increased.

After coding testing and debugging again and again this programme (shown in Figure S3) was made which was installed in the dispenser devices used in this study. The delay times were set after about 100 trial and error tests so that the run-time of the pump is perfect to pump out the required amount of sanitizer.

2.4. Fabrication Process

The fabrication and placements of the components are shown in Figure 3. To maintain the device's stability, the pump was placed on the bottom surface of the container while the nozzle was placed at about ≤ half-height of the container's height to take the advantage of liquid flow driven by gravity. Otherwise, the sanitizer may not get the needed pressure and the pump might not pump out the desired amount of liquids. The LDR sensor is kept inside a box or cabinet that is open to one side. Such an arrangement helps to make the nonfunctioning of the sensor due to the interference of natural sunlight or light from other sources such as vehicles, lamp posts, etc. This is a typical drawback of commercially available sensor-based dispensers, and some dispensers have a limitation to be placed only indoors because of the interference from unwanted light and sound signals (if an ultrasound sensor is used). An indicator LED strip was placed above the nozzle. This acts as an instruction for the user when to remove his/her hands from the laser detection chamber. Moreover, a cutout was made beside the transparent container and a LED strip was attached to the container. This action may help the user or maintenance authority to know the sanitizer level.

Preparation of Hand Sanitizer

At present, alcohol-based hand rubs are the only known means for rapidly and effectively inactivating a wide array of potentially harmful microorganisms on hands [23–28]. To help the countries and healthcare facilities, the World Health Organization (WHO) has recommended formulations for local preparation of alcohol-based hand rubs to be used for hand hygiene. Logistic, economic, safety, cultural, and religious factors have all been carefully considered by WHO before recommending such formulations for use worldwide. Hand sanitizer used in the automated touchless hand sanitizer dispenser developed in this study was prepared strictly following the WHO recommended formulation and procedure for local production [1], as shown in Table 3. The choice of components for the WHO-recommended hand rub formulations takes into accounts the cost constraints and microbicidal activity.

Table 3. World Health Organization recommended formulations for local production of alcohol-based hand sanitizer.

Formulation	Required Ingredients (Starting % of Ingredient)	Concentrations in Final Product, % (v/v), (Final % of Ingredient)	Required Volume of Ingredients for 10-L Preparation, mL
1	(i). Ethanol 96%	80	8333
	(ii). Hydrogen peroxide 3%	0.125	417
	(iii). Glycerol 98	1.45	145
	(iv). Sterile distilled water or boiled cold water	—	1105
2	(i). Isopropanol 99.8%	75	7515
	(ii). Hydrogen peroxide 3%	0.125	417
	(iii). Glycerol 98%	1.45	145
	(iv). Sterile distilled water or boiled cold water	—	1923

The required volume of ingredients (isopropyl alcohol, hydrogen peroxide and glycerol) was calculated using the following equation:

$$\text{Volume of starting ingredient required, (mL)} = \frac{(Final\ \%\ of\ ingredient)(Final\ volume\ of\ preparation)}{Starting\ \%\ of\ ingredient} \quad (9)$$

Note: when the concentration of alcohol (e.g., ethanol or isopropyl alcohol) in the starting ingredient is not exact, the calculation should be adjusted accordingly to ensure a final concentration of at least 80% ethanol or 75% isopropyl alcohol.

Hand sanitizer for the dispenser developed in this study was prepared as of formulation 2, though both of the formulations can be followed depending on the availability of ingredients in the local market. By using a measuring cylinder, an amount of 7515 mL isopropyl alcohol (99.8%), 417 mL hydrogen peroxide (3%), and 145 mL glycerol (98%) were poured into a precleaned plastic bottle to prepare 10-L sanitizer. The bottle was then topped up with sterile distilled or cold boiled water to make a total volume of 10-L. The screw cap was placed on the bottle as soon as possible in order to prevent evaporation. The solution was then mixed thoroughly by shaking gently. An alcoholmeter was used to control the isopropyl alcohol concentration of the final solution. The concentration of hydrogen peroxide was measured by the titrimetric method (oxidation-reduction reaction by iodine in acidic conditions). The absence of microbial contamination (including spores) was checked by filtration, according to the European Pharmacopeia specifications [26]. National safety guidelines and local legislation were strictly followed in the purchase, transportation and storage of ingredients, and the final product.

3. Working Principle of the Dispenser

At first, the device should be plugged in using a 12 V AC-DC adapter. Then the process will automatically start to run without any human interaction. The functionality of this dispenser device is simple. Whenever the user puts his/her hand inside the laser detection chamber, the laser light is distracted (or intensity of light is reduced) due to the opaque media; human—hand. As a consequence, the voltage gain from the LDR sensor increases and the current flow through the LDR photoresistor decreases. Whenever the voltage gain exceeds the threshold value, the microcontroller acts according to the inserted program and sends a command to the motor driver to operate the pump and the indicator LEDs.

In the working algorithm, a delay time was set before the microcontroller passes the trigger signal to run the pump. This initiative was taken to reduce the wastage of the liquid sanitizer in case of accidental disruption of the laser light signal. After the pump runs for a preprogrammed time, it turns off automatically and stops the flow of sanitizer. Then the process delays for a limited time (or the system becomes refreshed within a short time). Following the system revitalization, the loop starts again, and the machine becomes ready for rapid action. A delay time was also set between two consecutive full operations of the dispensing system, which also helps to reduce the wastage of sanitizer.

A cutaway was included by which one can observe the sanitizer liquid level inside the container and refill whenever needed. For refill and maintenance purposes, a portion of the upper surface of the device was made foldable at about 120° angle. Two probes were inserted inside the container. These probes act as the sanitizer level indicator by which the microcontroller can check whether the liquid level is high or low. Whenever the sanitizer level goes down, the connection between two probes gets disconnected and it lets the microcontroller know that the sanitizer level is low.

The running pump indicator LED strip is used to indicate that the pump is running and also it acts as an indication for users not to remove their hands from the chamber while the pump is still running. This initiative is also for reducing the wastage and also ensuring that the user gets the necessary amount of sanitizer needed to perfectly sanitize his/her hands. This indicator LED strip also indicates the low sanitizer level by blinking again and again, which is introduced in the code and also in the flowchart. As a result, the user may instantly know if there is sufficient sanitizer inside the container or not.

4. Results and Discussion

Deployment and Performance Analysis of the Device

A total of 20 units of fabricated devices, were deployed in four different metropolises in Bangladesh, and these regions have a clear variation in weather conditions. Figure 5 demonstrates the geographical locations of Bangladesh where the dispenser devices were deployed. Specifically, in each metropolis, several public locations such as hospitals, roadside bus stands, tea-stalls, varsity premises, etc., were chosen to deploy the devices. A list of the indoor and outdoor locations (where the devices were deployed) together with the GPS coordinates is shown in Table 4. These devices were deployed in the first week of June 2020, and their performances were analyzed from one to four months. Most of the deployed devices, that were fabricated according to the proposed design in this study, have shown an expected performance under the monitoring period.

Among 20 units of the dispenser devices, two units were found malfunctioned, another two units showed minor malfunctioning after a monitoring period of 1 month.

It was found that either the LDR sensor or the laser was damaged in the malfunctioned units. On the other hand, the disconnection of wires was observed in the minor malfunctioning units which could be the result of a transport problem or accidental shake or vibrations. For further confirmation of the reasons of malfunctioning, the malfunctioned units were analyzed by disassembling and reassembling the whole device. However, a number of external factors such as temperature, humidity, rainfall, UV index were identified as responsible for the damage of the sensor and laser light in the malfunctioned units. Analytics of these factors, particularly temperature and humidity are shown in Figures 5 and 6, respectively.

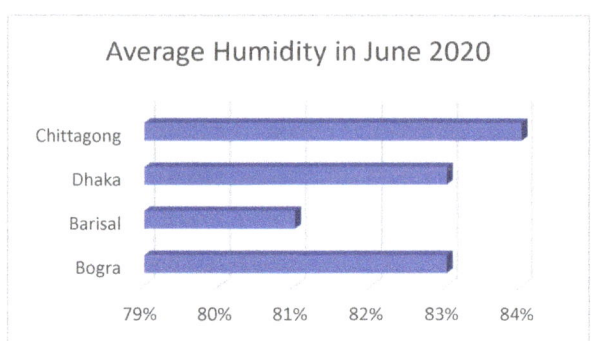

Figure 5. Average humidity comparison chart in June 2020.

Table 4. Deployment of the fabricated hand sanitizer dispenser units in various major cities in Bangladesh.

Deployed Locations	Address	GPS Coordinates	Number of Machines	Placement Environment	Observed Working Condition
Shaheed Ziaur Rahman Medical College	Bogra City Bypass, Bogura 5800	24°49′40.6″ N 89°21′10.8″ E	1	Indoor	Working
Mohammad Ali Hospital	01 Sherpur Rd, Bogura 5800	24°50′08.2″ N 89°22′27.0″ E	1	Indoor	Working
Choumatha Markaj Jame Masjid	C & B Rd, Bhanga-Barisal Hwy, Barishal 8200	22°42′02.9″ N 90°21′11.4″ E	1	Outdoor	Malfunctioned
Chittagong Medical College Hospital	57 K.B. Fazlul Kader Rd, Chattogram 4203	22°21′33.7″ N 91°49′50.6″ E	8	Four Indoor Four Outdoor	Working One unit minor malfunction
Nagar Bhaban	Batali Hill, Tiger Pass, Chattogram	22°20′39.9″ N 91°48′51.3″ E	2	Indoor	Working
GEC Circle Bus Stop	GEC More, Chattogram	22°21′32.7″ N 91°49′16.5″ E	1	Outdoor	Minor malfunction
Askar Ali Jame Masjid	Gundip, Anowara, Chattogram	22°20′22.1″ N 91°84′33.1″ E	1	Outdoor	Working
Sadar Thana Bogura	Bogura	24°51′01.6″ N 89°22′22.1″ E	1	Indoor	Working
Satmatha Traffic Police Box	Park Rd, Bogra	24°50′50.8″ N 89°22′21.3″ E	1	Outdoor	Malfunctioned
Chatori Choumohoni Bazar	Gundip, Anowara, Chattogram	22°23′27.4″ N 91°87′18.1″ E	1	Indoor	Working
Bangladesh Awami League Central Office	23 Bangabandhu Ave, Dhaka	23°43′36.3″ N 90°24′40.4″ E	2	Indoor	Working

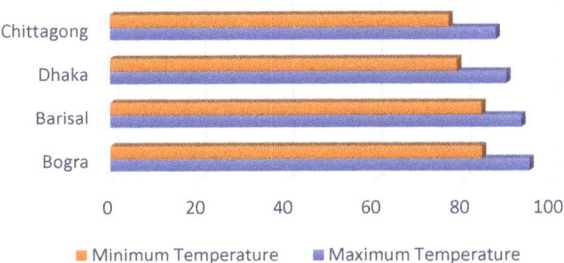

Figure 6. Maximum and minimum temperatures of the four districts in June 2020.

Figure 6 shows the maximum and minimum of temperature of the studied region with the following order Chittagong < Dhaka < Barisal < Bogra, while the humidity of the studied regions show an order of Barisal < Bogra < Dhaka < Chittagong (see in Figure 5).

It can be assumed that the performance of the photoresistor and the laser was affected by the temperature and humidity. The two malfunctioned units (that were deployed outdoors) were found in Barisal and Bogra. Since these two cities show relatively higher temperature, it can be assumed that the LDR sensor or the laser was damaged because of higher daytime temperature or excessive sunlight. On the other hand, the two semi malfunctioned units were found in Chittagong city where they were deployed in the outdoor environment. Since a greater value of humidity was found in this city, such a high humidity might cause the partial malfunctioning of the devices via dampening the sensor surface which prevented the laser to penetrate. Excessive dust can also be a reason for the partial malfunctioning. These assumptions are based on the fact that all dispenser units that were deployed in the indoor environment showed smooth functioning even after four months of deployment. It is thus assumed that the devices that were deployed in the outdoor environment and showed a partial or full malfunction were because of either the laser and LDR damage or affected due to the excessive dust, temperature, or humidity.

A review of literature revealed that numerous dispenser devices of various designs and sensing techniques are available in the market. However, all of these devices are rather expensive for the general population, especially for the people of the third world countries where a great portion of the total population are living under the poverty line. However, in order to perform a cost-effective analysis, the commonly used automated dispenser devices are listed in Table 5.

The prices shown in Table 5 were taken from different online shopping platforms like amazon.com and Aliexpress which are accessible to most of the countries in the world. After a thorough analysis of the online market prices, the commercial dispensers show a price range from USD 29 to 180, where our fabricated dispenser shows a maximum cost of only around USD 25. As this device is made of components that are available in almost every country at a very low price, mostly available on online sites, it is helpful for normal people to make a dispenser of their own. The present device can be made more cost-effective if the Arduino and motor driver circuits are replaced by a custom-made circuit using a relay instead of a microcontroller.

Table 5. Available dispenser devices name sensor power price.

Name	Price in (USD)	Sensor	Power Consumption/Cycle (W) $P = VI$
Bremmer Hand Sanitizer Dispenser Wall Mounted (1000 mL)	73.0583 Approx.	Infrared sensor	4 AA dry cell batteries. (1.5 V–0.5 Amp) 3 W
Zurio Automatic Hand Sanitizer Dispenser Wall Mount (450 mL)	59.99	Infrared sensor	12 V–0.5 A 6 W
JS LifeStyle Automatic Hand Sanitizer Dispenser (1000 mL)	29.99	Infrared sensor	3 AA battery (1.5 V–0.5 A) 2.25 W
Luxtonusa Automatic Hand Sanitizer Dispenser (500 mL)	179.95	Motion activated sensor	4 C-sized battery (1.5 V–3.8 A) 22.8 W
CasaTimo Automatic Touchless Hand Sanitizer Dispenser (450 mL)	35.99	Motion activated sensor	4 AA dry cell batteries. (1.5 V–0.5 Amp) 3 W
Safeline 360 Automatic Sanitizer/soap Dispenser (1000 mL)	59	Infrared sensor	4 AA dry cell batteries. (1.5 V–0.5 Amp) 3 W
Guukar Automatic Soap Dispenser Hand Sanitizer (500 mL)	41.99	Infrared sensor	4 AA dry cell batteries. (1.5 V–0.5 Amp) 3 W
Kent Auto Hand Sanitizer Dispenser (12,000 mL)	161.846 Approx.	Infrared sensor	Input: 230 V AC 24 V DC–1.5 A Total rated Consumption: 40 W
SaniQuick Touch Free Soap and Sanitizer Dispenser (3200 mL)	155.102 Approx.	Ultrasonic sensor	Input: 220 V AC

Most of these dispensing devices are operated based on AA batteries. However, since these batteries discharge faster, they need to be changed quite frequently which adds extra expense. To minimize such expenses and also to ensure a constant good performance, a 12 V–1 A AC to DC adapter was used in our fabricated device. Compared to the dispenser from KENT and SaniQuick, the present device consumes much less power (only 12 W/cycle) without sacrificing an equal graded performance. Table 5 shows that most of the automated sanitizing devices do not use a specific pump rather they are operated by a DC volt battery. However, as these devices rely on gravity, the mechanical pumping system becomes malfunctioning after a certain time of use because of "Buoyant force" and "Capillary force". Moreover, to take the advantage of gravity, these devices need to be set only at a position perpendicular to the ground.

Almost all of these devices used a custom-made valve to control the flow of the sanitizer; the working principle of this valve is mainly based on the gravitational pull. As a result, sometimes these devices face some leakage issues which can be avoided in the proposed designed dispenser as it is partially dependent on gravity but totally dependent on the pump.

The commercial devices (shown in Table 5) are using two types of sensors—infrared (IR) and ultrasound sensors. In general, the IR sensors show better accuracy than ultrasonic sensors. However, the IR sensors show some drawbacks like "Reading effects" by the infrared radiation of the sun light [29]. As a result, the IR sensor-based sanitizer dispensers cannot be deployed in an outdoor environment or in places having bright sunlight. On the other hand, to understand the effectiveness of our dispenser device compared to the ultrasound sensors, a real-time experiment was performed using the same experimental setup in this study. About 500 trials were recorded and after analyzing the results of the trial the outcome is shown in Figure 7.

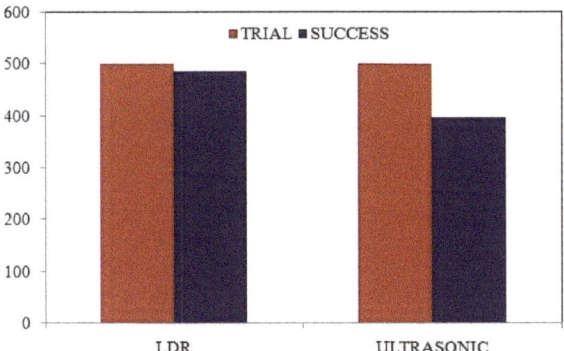

Figure 7. Comparison of trial-based success rate: (1) LDR sensor, (2) ultrasonic sensor.

Both devices with the LDR sensor and ultrasound sensor were placed in a crowded bus station (GEC Circle Bus Stop; 22°21′32.7″ N, 91°49′16.5″ E). From the column chart shown in Figure 7, it is crystal clear that for outdoor use, the ultrasonic sensor has shown underperformance compared to the current device of the laser detection system with an LDR sensor. One of the main drawbacks of the ultrasound sensor is that it provides garbage readings from different sound sources named the "Reading effect" [29]. As a result, the device sometimes runs automatically even if there is no user, consequently wasting the sanitizing material and making a mess underneath the device.

In the present device, the use of laser detection by an LDR sensor helps to avoid the reading effects typically found in the ultrasonic sensor. The LDR sensor is placed inside a 7 cm tall cabinet so that the reflected sunlight or other light sources cannot disturb the performance of the device. Moreover, the default delay time between two working cycles is lower in the case of LDR than the ultrasonic. As a result, LDR sensors have higher response frequency and lower delay time. In the present device, the volume of the container is 1000 mL. Since an approximate amount of 1 mL sanitizer is dispensed through the nozzle in an operation cycle, therefore 1 L of the sanitizing material is sufficient to serve about 1000 people.

5. Conclusions

In this study, a novel design of an automated hand sanitizer dispenser was demonstrated. The components needed for the device fabrication were described in detail. The circuit diagram was discussed, which clarifies the connection between the components with the microcontroller circuit (Arduino UNO). The piping conditions were shown and described accordingly. The relevant diagrams and components of the original device were presented in sequential order for a better understanding of the device fabrication process/model. Arduino IDE was used to input the program into the microcontroller. The algorithm used in this device was described with a flowchart to depict the functionality of the dispenser. A comparison was made to assess the effectiveness of the current LDR sensor with the ultrasonic and IR sensor which are generally used for commercial purposes. Based on this study, our fabricated device shows the following advantages:

- Superior performances for indoor use;
- Consumes low power; while in standby mode it consumes only 0.05 mA, and during the operating cycle it consumes about 12 V and 0.5 A;
- Cheap readymade components like Arduino Uno, L298 motor driver, 5 V laser, 5 mm LDR are used. As a result, this device can be made at a low cost with a price range from about USD 20 to 25;
- LDR sensor is more efficient to be used for proximity sensing than ultrasonic sensor in the case of the outdoor use of this dispenser.

The automatic touchless hand sanitizer device demonstrated in this study is expected to play a key role in contactless hand disinfection in public places and reduce the spread of infectious diseases in society.

Supplementary Materials: The following are available online at https://www.mdpi.com/article/10.3390/healthcare9040445/s1, Figure S1: 3D isometric view with parameters, Figure S2: Schematic of the dispenser circuit, Figure S3: The coding of the dispenser according to the algorithm.

Author Contributions: Conceptualization, A.D., A.B., M.U.K. and K.S.A.-m.; methodology, A.D.; software, A.D. and A.B.; validation, A.D., A.B., M.U.K. and K.S.A.-m.; formal analysis, A.D.; investigation, M.A.M., A.D. and A.B.; resources, A.D. and A.B.; data curation, M.A.M. and J.A.; writing—original draft preparation, A.D.; writing—review and editing, M.U.K.; visualization, A.D., A.B. and M.A.M.; supervision, M.U.K. and K.S.A.-m.; project administration, A.D.; funding acquisition, K.S.A.-m. All authors have read and agreed to the published version of the manuscript.

Funding: This work was funded by Deanship of Scientific Research at Princess Nourah Bint Abdulrahman University, through the Fast-track Research Funding (FRF) Program (grant no. 1000-ftfp-20).

Acknowledgments: The authors greatly acknowledge the contributions (from logistics to device deployment and data collection from various places in the country) made by Robo Mechatronics Association, CUET. Special thanks go to the members of this association who collected the data from across the country.

Conflicts of Interest: The authors declare no conflict of interest.

Nomenclature

V	Fluid velocity (m/s)
P	Fluid pressure (N/m^2)
g	Gravitational acceleration (m/s^2)
γ	Specific weight (N/m^3)
Z	Potential energy per unit weight (J/kg)
Q	Volumetric flow rate (m^3/s)
r	Radius (m)
ΔH	The head imparted to liquid by the pump (m)
H	Height (m)
V_0	Voltage at A0 pin of Arduino (Volt)
R1	10 kΩ resistance
R2	Resistance value of LDR (kΩ)

References

1. World Health Organization. *WHO Guidelines on Hand Hygiene in Health Care. First Global Patient Safety Challenge Clean Care Is Safer Care. World Alliance for Patient Safety*; WHO: Geneva, Switzerland, 2009.
2. Pittet, D.; Allegranzi, B.; Boyce, J. World Health Organization world alliance for patient safety first global patient safety challenge core group of experts. The World Health Organization guidelines on hand hygiene in health care and their consensus recommendations. *Infect. Control Hosp. Epidemiol.* **2009**, *30*, 611–622. [CrossRef] [PubMed]
3. White, C.; Kolble, R.; Carlson, R.; Lipson, N.; Dolan, M.; Ali, Y.; Cline, M. The effect of hand hygiene on illness rate among students in university residence halls. *Am. J. Infect. Control* **2003**, *31*, 364–370. [CrossRef]
4. Ehrenkranz, N.J.; Alfonso, B.C. Failure of bland soap handwash to prevent hand transfer of patient bacteria to urethral catheters. *Infect. Control Hosp. Epidemiol.* **1991**, *12*, 654–662. [CrossRef] [PubMed]
5. Fournier, A.K.; Berry, T.D. Effects of response cost and socially-assisted interventions on hand-hygiene behavior of university students. *Behav. Soc. Issues* **2012**, *21*, 152–164. [CrossRef]
6. Eiref, S.D.; Leitman, I.M.; Riley, W. Hand sanitizer dispensers and associated hospital-acquired infections: Friend or fomite? *Surg. Infect.* **2012**, *13*, 137–140. [CrossRef] [PubMed]
7. Würtz, R.; Moye, G.; Jovanovic, B. Handwashing machines, handwashing compliance, and potential for cross-contamination. *Am. J. Infect. Control* **1994**, *22*, 228–230. [CrossRef]
8. Bal, M.; Abrishambaf, R. A system for monitoring hand hygiene compliance based-on Internet-of-Things. In Proceedings of the IEEE International Conference on Industrial Technology (ICIT), Toronto, ON, Canada, 22–25 March 2017; pp. 1348–1353.
9. Rabeek, S.M.; Norman, A.; Je, M.; Raja, M.K.; Peh, R.F.; Dempsey, M.K. A reliable handwash detector for automated hand hygiene documentation and reminder system in hospitals. In *The 15th International Conference on Biomedical Engineering 2014*; Springer: Cham, Switzerland, 2014; pp. 892–895.

10. Zivich, P.N.; Huang, W.; Walsh, A.; Dutta, P.; Eisenberg, M.; Aiello, A.E. Measuring office workplace interactions and hand hygiene behaviors through electronic sensors: A feasibility study. *PLoS ONE* **2021**, *16*, e0243358. [CrossRef]
11. Karn, A.; Kanchi, R.; Deo, S.S.; Acres, E. Design and development of an automated monitored hand hygiene system to curb infection spread in institutional settings during COVID-19 Pandemic. In Proceedings of the International Conference on Advances in the Field of Health, Safety, Fire, Environment & Allied Sciences (HSFEA 2020), Dehradun, India, 18–19 December 2020.
12. Patra, R.; Bhattacharya, M.; Mukherjee, S. IoT-based computational frameworks in disease prediction and healthcare management: Strategies, challenges, and potential. In *IoT in Healthcare and Ambient Assisted Living*; Marques, G., Bhoi, A.K., de Albuquerque, V.H.C., Hareesha, K.S., Eds.; Springer: Singapore, 2021; pp. 17–41.
13. Nair, S.; Scurtu, I.C.; Hudișteanu, S.V. 10. Integrated health monitoring & disinfecting system for organizations and societies. In Proceedings of the International Conference Building Services and Energy Efficiency, Iasi, Romania, 2–3 July 2020; pp. 104–119.
14. Hong, T.S.; Bush, E.C.; Hauenstein, M.F.; Lafontant, A.; Li, C.; Wanderer, J.P.; Ehrenfeld, J.M. A hand hygiene compliance check system: Brief communication on a system to improve hand hygiene compliance in hospitals and reduce infection. *J. Med. Syst.* **2015**, *39*, 1–4. [CrossRef] [PubMed]
15. Chowdhury, B.; De, T. An Internet of Things Assisted Smart Hand Sanitizer with Health Monitoring System Help to Reduce Rapid Spread of COVID-19. Available online: https://easychair.org/publications/preprint/nLwv (accessed on 19 March 2021).
16. Baslyman, M.; Rezaee, R.; Amyot, D.; Mouttham, A.; Chreyh, R.; Geiger, G. Towards an RTLS-based hand hygiene notification system. *Procedia Comput. Sci.* **2014**, *37*, 261–265. [CrossRef]
17. Rojo, M.G.; Sy, J.B.; Calibara, E.R.; Comendador, A.V.; Degife, W.; Sisay, A. Non-contact temperature reader with sanitizer dispenser (NCTRSD). *Int. J. Sci. Res. Publ.* **2020**, *10*, 583–593. [CrossRef]
18. Srihari, M.M. Self-activating sanitizer with battery imposed system for cleansing hands. In Proceedings of the 2nd International Conference on Inventive Research in Computing Applications (ICIRCA), Coimbatore, India, 15–17 July 2020; pp. 1102–1105.
19. Lee, J.; Lee, J.-Y.; Cho, S.-M.; Yoon, K.-C.; Kim, Y.J.; Kim, K.G. Design of automatic hand sanitizer system compatible with various containers. *Healthc. Inform. Res.* **2020**, *26*, 243–247. [CrossRef] [PubMed]
20. Eddy, Y.; Mohammed, M.N.; Daoodd, I.I.; Bahrain, S.H.; Al-Zubaidi, S.; Al-Sanjary, O.I.; Sairah, A.K. 2019 Novel Coronavirus Disease (Covid-19): Smart contactless hand sanitizer-dispensing system using IoT based robotics technology. *Rev. Argent. Clin. Psicol.* **2020**, *29*, 215–220. [CrossRef]
21. Çengel, Y.A.; Cimbala, J.M. *Fluid Mechanics: Fundamentals and Applications*; McGraw-Hill Education: New York, NY, USA, 2018.
22. Atmel. 8-bit AVR Microcontrollers. ATmega328/P. 2016.
23. Pittet, D.; Hugonnet, S.; Harbarth, S.; Mourouga, P.; Sauvan, V.; Touveneau, S.; Perneger, T.V. Effectiveness of a hospital-wide programme to improve compliance with hand hygiene. *Lancet* **2000**, *356*, 1307–1312. [CrossRef]
24. Larson, E.L.; Eke, P.I.; Laughon, B.E. Efficacy of alcohol-based hand rinses under frequent-use conditions. *Antimicrob. Agents Chemother.* **1986**, *30*, 542–544. [CrossRef]
25. Larson, E.L.; Aiello, A.E.; Bastyr, J.; Lyle, C.; Stahl, J.; Cronquist, A.; Lai, L.; Della-Latta, P. Assessment of two hand hygiene regimens for intensive care unit personnel. *Crit. Care Med.* **2001**, *29*, 944–951. [CrossRef] [PubMed]
26. Widmer, A.F. Replace hand washing with use of a waterless alcohol hand rub? *Clin. Infect. Dis.* **2000**, *31*, 136–143. [CrossRef] [PubMed]
27. Maury, E.; Alzieu, M.; Baudel, J.L.; Haram, N.; Barbut, F.; Guidet, B.; Offenstadt, G. Availability of an alcohol solution can improve hand disinfection compliance in an intensive care unit. *Am. J. Respir. Crit. Care Med.* **2000**, *162*, 324–327. [CrossRef] [PubMed]
28. Bischoff, W.E.; Reynolds, T.M.; Sessler, C.N.; Edmond, M.B.; Wenzel, R.P. Handwashing compliance by health care workers: The impact of introducing an accessible, alcohol-based hand antiseptic. *Arch. Intern. Med.* **2000**, *160*, 1017–1021. [CrossRef] [PubMed]
29. Adarsh, S.; Kaleemuddin, S.M.; Bose, D.; Ramachandran, K.I. Performance comparison of Infrared and Ultrasonic sensors for obstacles of different materials in vehicle/robot navigation applications. *IOP Conf. Ser. Mater. Sci. Eng.* **2016**, *149*, 012141. [CrossRef]

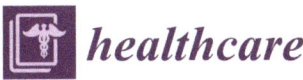

Article

Knowledge, Protective Behaviors and Risk Perception of COVID-19 among Dental Students in India: A Cross-Sectional Analysis

Kavita Batra [1,*], Yashashri Urankar [2], Ravi Batra [3], Aaron F. Gomes [4], Meru S [5] and Pragati Kaurani [6]

1. Office of Research, School of Medicine, University of Nevada, Las Vegas, NV 89102, USA
2. Community Health Centers of South-Central Texas, Gonzales, TX 78629, USA; UrankarY@chcsct.com
3. Department of Information Technology, Coforge Ltd., Atlanta, GA 30338, USA; ravi.batra@coforgetech.com
4. Department of Periodontology and Oral Implantology, Uttaranchal Dental and Medical Research Institute, Dehradun 248140, India; aarongomes@hotmail.com
5. Department of Oral Medicine and Radiology, Uttaranchal Dental and Medical Research Institute, Dehradun 248140, India; drmeru@gmail.com
6. Department of Prosthodontics, Mahatma Gandhi Dental College and Hospital, Jaipur 302022, India; drpragatikaurani@rediffmail.com
* Correspondence: Kavita.batra@unlv.edu

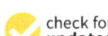

Citation: Batra, K.; Urankar, Y.; Batra, R.; Gomes, A.F.; S, M.; Kaurani, P. Knowledge, Protective Behaviors and Risk Perception of COVID-19 among Dental Students in India: A Cross-Sectional Analysis. *Healthcare* **2021**, *9*, 574. https://doi.org/10.3390/healthcare9050574

Academic Editor: Pedram Sendi

Received: 14 April 2021
Accepted: 11 May 2021
Published: 13 May 2021

Publisher's Note: MDPI stays neutral with regard to jurisdictional claims in published maps and institutional affiliations.

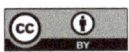

Copyright: © 2021 by the authors. Licensee MDPI, Basel, Switzerland. This article is an open access article distributed under the terms and conditions of the Creative Commons Attribution (CC BY) license (https://creativecommons.org/licenses/by/4.0/).

Abstract: Objective: This study's objective was to examine the knowledge, performance in practicing protective behaviors, and risk perception of Coronavirus disease-19 (COVID-19) among dental students of India. Methods: A web-based cross-sectional survey was conducted from 10–30 August 2020, involving 381 dental students that were enrolled at the Uttaranchal Dental and Medical Research Institute in India. A web-based structured questionnaire assessed the COVID-19 related knowledge, protective behaviors, and risk perception performance. The independent-samples-t and analysis of variance tests were used to analyze the differences in knowledge, protective behaviors, and perception across the groups. Results: Of the dental students surveyed, 83% had adequate knowledge of COVID-19, and nearly 80% followed appropriate practices regarding COVID-19. The COVID-19 related risk perception was higher among females as compared to males. COVID-19 related knowledge was significantly correlated with preventive behaviors ($r = 0.18$; $p < 0.01$) and risk perception ($r = 0.10$; $p < 0.05$). We found a high score of COVID-19 related knowledge and precautionary behaviors and moderate risk perception among students. Conclusions: Knowledge and protective behaviors towards infectious diseases, such as COVID-19, have clinical applications in developing educational and formal training programs to promote adherence to the infection control practices among dental students. Clinical significance: The findings of this study will inform policymakers to emphasize on effective risk communication. Dental institutions can incorporate infection control modules in the current curriculum, thereby making future dental professionals capable of performing effective infection control management in the clinical settings. This is critical in improving their knowledge of infection control practices to minimize the risk of nosocomial infections.

Keywords: COVID-19; dental precautions; dental students; India; infection control; knowledge; perception; survey

1. Introduction

The World Health Organization (WHO), on 11 March 2020, declared novel Coronavirus disease (COVID-19) a pandemic caused by a viral strain, named as SARS-CoV-2 [1]. There are more than 104,370,550 confirmed cases globally, and 2,271,180 deaths were reported as of 5 February 2021, while writing this manuscript [1]. Currently, there are nearly 10,814,656 confirmed COVID-19 cases in India alone [2]. COVID-19 reported to be highly contagious when compared to its previous predecessors [3], and it possesses a relatively higher reproductive number (R_0), ranging from 2 to 4. In other words, on an average, a

COVID-19 infected individual can transmit the virus or infect 2–4 individuals during the course of time [3]. The primary mode of transmission of COVID-19 is person-to-person via respiratory droplets either inhaled or through contact, with the typical incubation period ranging from 2–14 days [4–6]. Globally, regulatory bodies provided infection control guidelines and standard operating procedures to curb the COVID-19 transmission in the dental settings [7]. These guidelines were related to clinical workspace, the use of personal protective equipment (PPE), disposal of PPE, disinfection of surfaces, and operatory to minimize the COVID-19 transmission. In March, 2020, the Dental Council of India (DCI) issued its first set of advisory, which were later updated during the course of pandemic [8].

To minimize the transmission of the virus, public health organizations have recommended standard preventive measures, including the use of face coverings, practicing social distancing, maintaining hand hygiene, and limiting contact with infected individuals [9,10]. These public health actions are necessary to minimize the spread; however, challenges that are associated with behavior adoption can pose significant barriers [11]. Furthermore, the dissemination of a vast amount of unreliable and unclear information on social media can complicate containment measures of COVID-19 and induce panic among the public [11–13].

Dental professionals and dental students are especially vulnerable due to their proximity to symptomatic or asymptomatic patients and their oral fluids [14,15]. According to one Japan-based study, the SARS-CoV-2 virus was found in 11 out of 12 COVID-19 patients [15]. The aerosols and droplets that were generated through dental procedures, the possible inhalation of airborne microorganisms, and direct or indirect contact with contaminated instruments are the potential routes of transmission in the dental care settings [16–18]. Previous studies that were conducted in Iran, Peru, and India reported insufficient knowledge of infection control practices among dental professionals [19–22]. The adherence to protective behaviors among healthcare students is enormously crucial among countries with healthcare workforce scarcity [23]. According to the National Health Profile, India has one doctor per 10,000 population of patients instead of the WHO recommendation of having one doctor per 1000 population of patients [11]. The apparent deficiency in the number of healthcare workforce can be potentially offset by dental workforce [23]. India achieved a higher dentist-to-patient ratio of 1:5000 as compared to WHO recommended ratio of 1:7500, with the rural–urban distribution being uneven [11]. In times of a healthcare crisis, dental professionals/students can be assigned hospital-based responsibilities to assist in the response efforts and gain practical experience to handle such future outbreaks [23]. In this context, knowledge regarding the prevention and control of COVID-19 transmission is essential for dental professionals/students to improve the preparedness and response actions. Informing future dentists about a pandemic disease at the initial learning stage is critical. Thus, they will be better equipped to play an active role in preventing and controlling disease during future outbreaks or spikes in the ongoing pandemic. Therefore, this study aimed to assess the knowledge, risk perception, and adherence to preventive behaviors among dental students regarding the COVID-19 pandemic.

2. Materials and Methods

2.1. Study Design and Study Participants

This descriptive, cross-sectional survey study was conducted from 10 August 2020 to 30 August 2020, among dental students in India. Full-time dental students (undergraduate, interns, and postgraduate), currently enrolled in any of the private, government, or deemed universities, who were of Indian nationality, were aged 18 years or above, had internet access, could provide informed consent, and comprehend English, were invited to participate in this survey. Part-time students, alumni, and those with no internet access and an inability to understand English were excluded from this study.

2.2. Ethical Consideration

The ethical approval was obtained from the institutional ethics committee (Uttaranchal Dental and Medical Research Institute [UDMRI], Mazri Grant, Dehradun, India., Ref. No. IEC/PA-02/2020, 8 August 2020). The ethics committee reviewed and approved this study protocol, participant information sheet (PIS), informed consent form, and the survey questionnaire. All of the study participants were requested to sign the informed consent to confirm their willingness to participate by answering an agree/disagree question. Informed consent included detailed information that was related to the aim and significance of the study so that participants could make an informed choice about whether to participate or withdraw at any time if he/she so wished. The participants who selected the "agree" option were directed to complete the self-administered questionnaire. All of the participants' anonymity was ensured, and no personal identifiers, including names, email IDs, and details of COVID-19 exposure, were collected. Only one response per Internet Protocol (IP) address was allowed.

2.3. Recruitment and Data Collection

This web-based survey was developed through Qualtrics (Provo, UT). The convenience sampling method was used for sample recruitment. The survey link was disseminated through emails and WhatsApp groups among the target student populations. The WhatsApp groups was otherwise used by faculty members to deliver notes, announcements, and lectures as part of a virtual instruction model that was recently implemented in response to the COVID-19 pandemic. The questionnaire was sent to 480 students, and 381 completed the survey. Therefore, the response rate was 80.2%.

2.4. Survey Instruments and Variables

The online survey questionnaire had a total of 33 questions and four sections: (1) demographic information; (2) COVID-19 related knowledge; (3) questions that were related to preventive behaviors for COVID-19; and, (4) questions to assess risk perception of COVID-19.

Demographics: the first section of the questionnaire contained six questions related to demographics, including gender, age, degree course, and COVID-19 education. These questions were developed based on previous literature [24,25].

COVID-19 related knowledge: we used 15 items questionnaire for assessing COVID-19 related knowledge. This tool has been validated by previous studies during historical outbreaks, such as Middle East Respiratory Syndrome (MERS) and Severe Acute Respiratory Syndrome (SARS), and has the reliability (Cronbach's α) of 0.72 with a content validity index of 0.95 [25,26]. This tool includes questions on the COVID-19 causes (three items); modes of transmission (two items); symptoms and latent period (two items); prevention, assessment, and treatment methods (seven items); and, guidelines for patient care (one item) [25,27]. These questions had possible responses of true/false/not sure options [25–27]. A correct answer was assigned one point, and an incorrect/unknown answer was assigned 0 points [25–27]. The total knowledge score ranged from 0 to 15, with a higher score [25–27] indicating a better knowledge of COVID-19.

Preventive behaviors for COVID-19: this tool was used to assess the performance rate for COVID-19-related preventive behaviors among participants. This tool has been previously used and validated by previous studies [25] on MERS. There was a total of nine items, of which five items were related to minimizing the use of public spaces, avoiding social gatherings, outdoor activities, and enclosed spaces, and minimizing contact with people showing cough symptoms, three items about practicing good hygiene, including handwashing, cleaning, and sanitization, and one item about talking with people about measures to take after COVID-19 infection [25,27]. The behavior (if practiced) was assigned 1 point, and 0 points were assigned if a behavior was not practiced by the participant. The total score ranged from 0–9; a high score was indicative of a high-performance rate [25,27]. The questionnaire has been validated and has a reliability index (Cronbach's α) of 0.77 [24–27].

Risk perception of COVID-19: COVID-19 related risk perception was conceptualized as the participant's fear of being infected with COVID-19. The scale of risk perception [25–27] had two items (i.e., 'I may be infected with COVID-19 more easily than others' and 'I am afraid to be infected with COVID-19'). Each item was assessed on a five-point scale from 1 (Never) to 5 (Always). The scale has been validated by previous studies [25–27], which were performed during SARS [26] and MERS [27] outbreaks.

2.5. Statistical Analysis

Participants' responses, from Qualtrics, were exported to Microsoft Excel (Microsoft Corporation, Richmond, WV, USA), and then imported to IBM SPSS version 26.0 (IBM Corp. Armonk, NY, USA). COVID-19 related knowledge, preventive practices, and risk perception were the quantitative variables in this study. Descriptive statistics, including the frequencies, proportions, mean, and standard deviations, were generated. Independent-samples- t-test and analysis of variance were utilized to analyze the differences in mean scores across different students' groups. The Pearson's correlations test was utilized to calculate the correlations among the variables. p-values less than 0.05 (two-sided) were considered to be statistically significant, and data were reported as 95% confidence intervals. The priori power analysis was conducted through G power (version 3.1) to ascertain the required sample size for a test with a predetermined alpha, beta (power), and Cohen's effect size conventions [28,29]. The sample size of n = 302 was considered to be appropriate after factoring in 20% incomplete entries or missing values.

3. Results

Sample Characteristics

A total of 381 responses were recorded during the survey period. The average time that was taken to complete the survey was 8.4 min. The demographic profile of the respondents shows that 268 (70.3%) respondents were females, and 79 (20.7%) were males (Table 1). The average age of the sample was 22.8 years (SD = 2.8 years). The majority of the participants were undergraduates (80%, n = 320), with nearly 48% (154 out of 320) being in the third and fourth year of the undergraduate dental program (Table 1). Approximately 64.8% participants had received some form of COVID-19 related education, and 50.7% of the COVID-19 related information was received from social media (Table 1). There were significant gender differences in the mean scores of knowledge and risk perception ($p < 0.05$). The mean knowledge scores were higher among male participants (M = 13.91, SD = 0.78) than females (M = 13.66, SD = 0.9), with a statistically significant mean difference, M = 0.25 95% CI [0.028, 0.46], $p = 0.04$, Table 1). Significant differences in the risk perception across gender were also noted ($p = 0.01$, Table 1). The mean score of risk perception was slightly higher (M = 3.0, SD = 1.0) among participants without prior COVID-19 education when compared to those who had some sort of education (M = 2.7, SD = 1.0), with a statistically significant mean difference, M = -0.30, 95% CI [-0.05, -0.55], $p = 0.02$, Table 1). There were no statistically significant differences found in the mean scores of preventive behaviors across any sample categories. The mean level of COVID-19-related knowledge was 83.0%. The COVID-19 knowledge item with the highest correct-answer rate (91.3%) was 'The first case of COVID-19 was diagnosed in Wuhan, China. (T)'. However, the items with the lowest correct answer rates were 'The disease can be treated by usual antiviral drugs. (F)' (45.4%) and 'Only during intubation, suction, bronchoscopy, and cardiopulmonary resuscitation, you have to wear an N95 mask (T)' (50.4%). The mean performance rate of COVID-related preventive behaviors was 79.9%. The behavior items with the highest performance rates were 'I reduced the use of public transportation' and 'I went shopping less frequently' and 'I reduced the use of closed spaces, such as library and theatre' (90.8%, Table 2). However, the items with relatively lower performance rates were 'I discussed, with my family and friends, what we should do if infected with COVID-19' (82.9%) and 'I increased the frequency of cleaning and disinfecting items that can be easily touched with hands (i.e., door handles and surfaces)' (86.3%). The total mean score of

COVID-19 related risk perception was 2·78 out of 5, and the score for fear of being infected with COVID-19 was 3.1 out of 5 (Table 3). COVID-19 related knowledge was significantly correlated with preventive behaviors ($r = 0.18$; $p < 0.01$) and risk perception ($r = 0.10$; $p < 0.05$). Besides, risk perception was significantly correlated with age ($r = 0.27$; $p < 0.01$; Table 4).

Table 1. Demographic characteristics of the study population (n = 381).

Variables	Characteristic	n (%)	Knowledge (Range: 0–100%) M ± SD	p-value	Preventive Behaviors (Range: 0–100%) M ± SD	p-value	Risk Perception (Range: 1–5) M ± SD	p-value
Gender	Male	79 (20.7)	13.91 ± 0.78	0.04 *	8.75 ± 0.55	0.27 **	2.48 ± 1.1	0.01 *
	Female	268 (70.3)	13.66 ± 0.94		8.82 ± 0.47		2.90 ± 1.0	
	Not reported	34 (9)	-		-		-	
Degree course	Undergraduate dental	320 (84)	13.68 ± 0.91	0.2 *	8.79 ± 0.50	0.8 *	2.7 ± 1.0	<0.001 *
	Post-graduate dental	33 (8.7)	13.88 ± 0.90		8.81 ± 0.54		3.6 ± 1.0	
	Not reported	28 (7.3)						
Received formal education about COVID-19	Yes	247 (64.8)	13.70 ± 0.87	0.1 *	8.83 ± 0.50	0.09 *	2.7 ± 1.0	0.02*
	No	102 (26.8)	13.69 ± 1.03		8.73 ± 0.51		3.0 ± 1.0	
	Not reported	32 (8.4)						
Source of education	Social media	193 (50.7)	13.72 ± 1.0	0.2 **	8.78 ± 0.52	0.4 **	2.7 ± 1.0	0.5 **
	TV/Radio	62 (16.3)	13.69 ± 1.0	-	8.82 ± 0.45	-	2.6 ± 1.0	-
	College	36 (9.4)	13.94 ± 0.9	-	8.83 ± 0.51	-	3.2 ± 1.1	-
	Newspapers	33 (8.7)	13.57 ± 0.75	-	8.76 ± 0.50	-	3.0 ± 1.0	-
	Others (Family/Friends)	29 (7.6)	13.43 ± 0.91	-	8.83 ± 0.40	-	2.8 ± 1.0	-
	Not reported	28 (7.3)						

* Independent-samples-*t*-test. ** Analysis of variance.

Table 2. Assessment of knowledge related to COVID-19 (n = 381).

	Items (True or False); Possible Range: (0.0–100.0%)	Correct Answer Rate (Range 0–100%)
1.	COVID-19 is a respiratory infection caused by a new species of coronavirus family. (T)	86.6
2.	The first case of COVID-19 was diagnosed in Wuhan, China. (T)	91.3
3.	The origin of COVID-19 is not clear, but it seems that it has been transmitted to humans by seafoods, snakes, or bats. (T)	83.2
4.	Its common symptoms are fever, cough, and shortness of breath, but nausea and diarrhea were reported rarely. (T)	87.6
5.	Its incubation period is up to 14 days with a mean of 5 days. (T)	88.7
6.	It can be diagnosed by PCR test on samples collected from nasopharyngeal and oropharyngeal discharge or from sputum and bronchial washing. (T)	86.6
7.	It is transmitted through respiratory droplets such as cough and sneeze. (T)	89.8
8.	It is transmitted through close contacts with an infected case (especially in family, crowded places and health centers). (T)	90.8
9.	The disease can be prevented through handwashing and personal hygiene. (T)	88.7
10.	A medical mask is useful to prevent the spread of respiratory droplets during coughing. (T)	89.5
11.	The disease can be prevented through no close contacts such as handshakes or kissing, not attending meetings and frequent hand disinfection. (T)	89.2
12.	All people in society should wear masks. (T)	87.4
13.	Only during intubation, suction, bronchoscopy and cardiopulmonary resuscitation, you have to wear N95 mask. (T)	50.4
14.	The disease can be treated by usual antiviral drugs. (F)	45.4
15.	If symptoms appear within 14 days from direct contact with a suspected case, the person should inquire at a nearby public health center. (T)	89.2
	Total	83.0

Table 3. Preventive behaviors and risk perception of COVID-19 (n = 381).

Items: Preventive Behaviors for COVID-19	Correct Answer Rate (Range 0–100%)
I canceled or postponed meetings with friends, eating out, and sport Events	89.5
I reduced the use of public transportation	90.8
I went shopping less frequently	90.8
I reduced the use of closed spaces, such as library and theatre	90.8
I avoided coughing around people as much as possible	89.2
I avoided places where many people gathered	90.0
I increased the frequency of cleaning and disinfecting items that can be easily touched with hands (i.e., door handles and surfaces)	86.3
I washed the hands more often than usual	89.5
I discussed, with my family and friends, what we should do if infected with COVID-19	82.9
Total	**79.9**
Risk Perception of COVID-19 (Possible Range: 1–5)	**M ± SD**
I may be infected with COVID-19 more easily than others	2.44 ± 1.25
I am afraid to be infected with COVID-19.	3.11 ± 1.30
Total	**2.78 ± 1.05**

M, mean, SD, Standard deviation, COVID-19, Coronavirus disease-2019.

Table 4. Correlation between COVID-19 knowledge, protective behaviors, risk perception and age (n = 381).

Variables	Knowledge	Preventive Behaviors	Risk Perception	Age in Years
Knowledge	1.00	-	-	-
Preventive behaviors	0.18 **	1.00	-	-
Risk perception	0.10 *	−0.03	1.00	-
Age in years	−0.08	0.03	0.27 *	1.00

* $p < 0.05$; ** $p < 0.01$.

4. Discussion

The current descriptive study assessed the knowledge, risk perception, and adherence to the protective behaviors of dental students in India regarding COVID-19. We found moderate levels of COVID-19 related knowledge (83.0%) and adherence to protective behaviors (79.9%) among the dental students. In our sample, nearly half (50.7%) of the study participants obtained COVID-19 education through social media, and only 9.4% reported obtaining the knowledge from college. These results were consistent with another Nigeria based study of undergraduate dental students [18]. Every three out of four students reported lack of formal COVID-19 related education or training in the college settings, as reported by a Turkish study [30]. This might be due to the lack of time available to the universities or colleges to design education programs focused on transmission-based infection control practices following the sudden invasion by the COVID-19 pandemic [11,16,25]. Transmission-based precautions differ from standard measures in providing additional guidance in controlling the spread of rapidly evolving pathogens, such as Coronavirus [31–33]. In addition, previous studies found that dental education in India emphasizes blood-borne infection control practices with limited training on the prevention and control of airborne or droplet infections [16]. The dental council of India published comprehensive infection control guidelines in 2009, which seem to be underutilized, even after a decade now [32]. In 2011, knowledge, attitudes, and practices of dental safety among 1874 dentists across eight countries were assessed and only 50% of participants reported utilizing standard infection control practices [33]. Therefore, this study underscores the need to revise the dental curriculum for developing a comprehensive module to teach effective transmission-based infection control practices to the students.

The study item with the highest scores of 91.3% was about the knowledge related to the origin of the COVID-19 pandemic. However, one item (i.e., 'disease could be treated by common antiviral drugs') had the lowest correct answer rates of 45.4%. This may be attributed to the rapidly evolving information that was related to the treatment of COVID-19 and surrounding controversies [34]. In this study, an 88.7% correct answer rate was found with the question that was related to the incubation period, which is greater than that reported in a Jordan based research (36.1%). This disparity may be due to the study period's difference; the Jordanian study was conducted in the early phases of the pandemic when epidemiological characteristics of the COVID-19 were not yet unfolded [35]. Consistent with previous reports [18,35,36], our study participants had a good knowledge of COVID-19 symptoms, which is essential for the early detection of suspected cases to take prompt actions. The performance rate to adhere to the protective behaviors was 79.9%, which was slightly higher than the 73.8% reported by a study conducted in China [37].

Inconsistent with a Nigeria-based study, our study found variations in the risk perceptions by gender [38]. The mean scores for risk perception about the COVID-19 were higher among female students than males (2.90 vs. 2.48, $p = 0.01$). The higher risk perception among females can be explained by their unrealistic perception, gender socialization, and awareness of health warnings [39–41]. Additionally, gender also predicted adherence to the protective behaviors, suggesting that females had a higher score of protective behaviors than males. These findings were consistent with the previous study [38]. The knowledge scores of females were lower than the males, and this finding was inconsistent with the other studies [37,42]. Our study found a higher score among postgraduate students than undergraduates, because clinical students rely more on science-based resources, such as the Ministry of Health rather than social media [43]. There were significant differences found in the COVID-19 knowledge and protective behaviors among clinical and preclinical students, and the results were consistent other studies that were conducted in Turkey, China, Saudi Arabia, Italy, and Nigeria [18,30,43–46]. The lower knowledge scores among undergraduate students highlight the need to refine the current dental curriculum, including infectious diseases epidemiology and control practices. This formal training of the preclinical students will help in increasing their understanding of the safety protocols. Students in the health sciences disciplines should acquire appropriate practical skills for infection control practices. Continuous education and assessment in the clinical setting may aid in improving the learning outcomes [47]. During the COVID-19 pandemic, the lack of practical training among students emerged as a concern, which can be addressed through new technological innovations [46–50]. Educators need to be trained for adopting new virtual platforms of teaching, which could be used in the future crisis. In addition, dental operatories need to be observed for the safety of patients as well as dental professionals [46–50]. In addition, future studies can be conducted to investigate the adherence of healthcare professionals with the recommended infection control practices.

Study Limitations

This investigation has some limitations. First, by the cross-sectional nature of this study, cause–effect relationships have not been studied. Second, this study's nonprobability sampling method may have introduced a selection bias as participants were approached via web-based platforms. Third, the sample was not nationally representative, and it was recruited from only the Northern region, limiting our ability to extrapolate our findings to the other dental institutions. Fourth, this study only assessed the general protective behaviors that were related to COVID-19, and it did not include any question related to the adoption of precautionary behaviors in dental clinics. Last, this study may encounter some degree of selection bias due to its cross-sectional design. Prospective studies can be designed to measure safety compliance in the dental practice to dental practice guidelines.

5. Conclusions

Our study indicated that dental students had sufficient knowledge regarding the COVID 19 pandemic. The students displayed responsible social behavior, which could be correlated to their level of knowledge on the pandemic. This study highlights the need to restructure the educational curriculum to prepare students to handle COVID-19 and future pandemics. This is critical in improving their knowledge of infection control practices to minimize the risk of nosocomial infections.

Author Contributions: Conceptualization, K.B. and R.B.; methodology, K.B.; software, R.B.; validation, K.B., R.B. and Y.U.; formal analysis, K.B. and R.B.; investigation, K.B., R.B. and Y.U.; resources, R.B., K.B., P.K., and Y.U.; data curation, A.F.G., M.S., K.B. and R.B.; writing—K.B., Y.U. and R.B.; Review and editing—All authors.; visualization, K.B.; supervision, A.F.G., M.S. and K.B.; project administration, K.B. All authors have read and agreed to the published version of the manuscript.

Funding: This research received no external funding.

Institutional Review Board Statement: The study was conducted according to the guidelines of the Declaration of Helsinki and approved by the Institutional Review Board (or Ethics Committee) of (Uttaranchal Dental and Medical Research Institute [UDMRI], Mazri Grant, Dehradun, India., Ref. No. IEC/PA-02/2020, 8 August 2020).

Informed Consent Statement: Informed consent was obtained from all subjects involved in the study.

Data Availability Statement: Data can be available from corresponding author upon request.

Conflicts of Interest: The authors declare no conflict of interest.

Abbreviations

COVID-19	Coronavirus disease-19
WHO	World Health Organization
PPE	Personal Protective Equipment
DCI	Dental Council of India
UDMRI	Uttaranchal Dental and Medical Research Institute
PIS	Participant Information Sheet
MERS	Middle East Respiratory Syndrome
SARS	Severe Acute Respiratory Syndrome
M	Mean
S.D	Standard Deviation

References

1. World Health Organization. WHO Coronavirus Disease (COVID-19) Dashboard. 2020. Available online: https://covid19.who.int/ (accessed on 5 February 2021).
2. Live Asia COVID-19 Statistics, Map and News [Internet]. Updated Every Minute! 2020. Available online: https://www.covid19.onl/region/asia (accessed on 5 February 2021).
3. Liu, Y.; Gayle, A.A.; Wilder-Smith, A.; Rocklöv, J. The reproductive number of COVID-19 is higher compared to SARS coronavirus. *J. Travel Med.* **2020**, *27*, taaa021. [CrossRef] [PubMed]
4. Abdel Wahed, W.Y.; Hefzy, E.M.; Ahmed, M.I.; Hamed, N.S. Assessment of Knowledge, Attitudes, and Perception of Health Care Workers Regarding COVID-19, A Cross-Sectional Study from Egypt. *J. Commun. Health* **2020**, *45*, 1242–1251. [CrossRef] [PubMed]
5. Rahman, H.S.; Aziz, M.S.; Hussein, R.H.; Othman, H.H.; Salih Omer, S.H.; Khalid, E.S.; Abdulrahman, N.A.; Amin, K.; Abdullah, R. The transmission modes and sources of COVID-19: A systematic review. *Int. J. Surg. Open* **2020**, *26*, 125–136. [CrossRef]
6. Singhal, T. A review of coronavirus disease-2019 (COVID-19). *Indian J. Pediatrics* **2020**, *87*, 281–286. [CrossRef] [PubMed]
7. Bescos, R.; Casas-Agustench, P.; Belfield, L.; Brookes, Z.; Gabaldón, T. Coronavirus Disease 2019 (COVID-19): Emerging and Future Challenges for Dental and Oral Medicine. *J. Dent. Res.* **2020**, *99*, 1113. [CrossRef]
8. Dental Council of India—Precautionary and Preventive Measures to Prevent Spread of Novel Coronavirus (COVID-19). Available online: https://dciindia.gov.in/Admin/NewsArchives/L.No._8855.PDF (accessed on 21 November 2020).
9. Centers for Disease Control and Prevention. Coronavirus Disease 2019 (COVID-19). 2020. Available online: https://www.cdc.gov/coronavirus/2019-ncov/index.html (accessed on 30 September 2020).
10. Ministry of Health & Family Welfare-Government of India. National health profile (NHP) of India-2019. 2020. Available online: https://www.cbhidghs.nic.in/showfile.php?lid=1147 (accessed on 12 October 2020).

11. Azlan, A.A.; Hamzah, M.R.; Sern, T.J.; Ayub, S.H.; Mohamad, E. Public knowledge, attitudes and practices towards COVID-19: A cross-sectional study in Malaysia. *PLoS ONE* **2020**, *15*, e0233668. [CrossRef]
12. Sharma, A. Covid-19 knowledge, attitude and practice among medical students. *Int. J. Sci. Res.* **2020**, *9*, 6–8. [CrossRef]
13. Ul Haq, N.; Hassali, M.A.; Shafie, A.A.; Saleem, F.; Farooqui, M.; Aljadhey, H. A cross sectional assessment of knowledge, attitude and practice towards Hepatitis B among healthy population of Quetta, Pakistan. *BMC Public Health* **2012**, *12*, 692. [CrossRef]
14. Li, G.; Chang, B.; Li, H.; Wang, R.; Li, G. Precautions in dentistry against the outbreak of corona virus disease 2019. *J. Infect. Public Health* **2020**, *13*, 1805–1810. [CrossRef] [PubMed]
15. Wang, K.K.; Tsang, O.T.; Yip, C.C.; Chan, K.H.; Wu, T.C.; Chun-Chan, J.M.; Leung, W.-S.; Thomas, S.-H.C.; Chris, Y.-C.C.; Darshana, H.K.; et al. Consistent Detection of 2019 Novel Coronavirus in Saliva. *Clin. Infect. Dis.* **2020**, *71*, 841–843. Available online: https://academic.oup.com/cid/article/71/15/841/5734265 (accessed on 12 October 2020).
16. Ghai, S. Are dental schools adequately preparing dental students to face outbreaks of infectious diseases such as COVID-19? *J. Dent. Educ.* **2020**, *84*, 631–633. [CrossRef]
17. Occupational Safety and Health Administration. Guidance on Preparing Workplaces for COVID-19. Available online: https://www.osha.gov/Publications/OSHA3990.pdf (accessed on 12 October 2020).
18. Umeizudike, K.A.; Isiekwe, I.G.; Fadeju, A.D.; Akinboboye, B.O.; Aladenika, E.T. Nigerian undergraduate dental students' knowledge, perception, and attitude to COVID-19 and infection control practices. *J. Dent. Educ.* **2021**, *85*, 187–196. [CrossRef]
19. Askarian, M.; Assadian, O. Infection control practices among dental professionals in Shiraz Dentistry School, Iran. *Arch. Iran. Med.* **2009**, *12*, 48–51.
20. Halboub, E.S.; Al-Maweri, S.A.; Al-Jamaei, A.A.; Tarakji, B.; Al-Soneidar, W.A. Knowledge, Attitudes, and Practice of Infection Control among Dental Students at Sana'a University, Yemen. *J. Int. Oral. Health* **2015**, *7*, 15–19.
21. Khubrani, A.; Albesher, M.; Alkahtani, A.; Alamri, F.; Alshamrani, M.; Masuadi, E. Knowledge and information sources on standard precautions and infection control of health sciences students at King Saud bin Abdulaziz University for Health Sciences, Saudi Arabia, Riyadh. *J. Infect. Public Health* **2018**, *11*, 546–549. [CrossRef] [PubMed]
22. Silva, O.; Palomino, S.; Robles, A.; Ríos, J.; Mayta-Tovalino, F. Knowledge, Attitudes, and Practices on Infection Control Measures in Stomatology Students in Lima, Peru. *J. Environ. Public Health* **2018**, *2018*, 8027130. [CrossRef]
23. Mahase, E. Covid-19: Portugal closes all medical schools after 31 cases confirmed in the country. *BMJ* **2020**, *368*, m986. [CrossRef] [PubMed]
24. Gautret, P.; Benkouiten, S.; Salaheddine, I.; Belhouchat, K.; Drali, T.; Parola, P.; Brouqui, P. Hajj pilgrim's knowledge about Middle East respiratory syndrome coronavirus, August to September 2013. *Eurosurveill* **2013**, *18*, 20604. [CrossRef] [PubMed]
25. Kim, J.S.; Choi, J.S. Middle East respiratory syndrome-related knowledge, preventive behaviours and risk perception among nursing students during outbreak. *J. Clin. Nurs.* **2016**, *25*, 2542–2549. [CrossRef]
26. Brug, J.; Aro, A.R.; Oenema, A.; de Zwart, O.; Richardus, J.H.; Bishop, G.D. SARS risk perception, knowledge, precautions, and information sources, the Netherlands. *Emerg. Infect. Dis.* **2004**, *10*, 1486–1489. [CrossRef]
27. Taghrir, M.H.; Borazjani, R.; Shiraly, R. COVID-19 and Iranian Medical Students; A Survey on Their Related-Knowledge, Preventive Behaviors and Risk Perception. *Arch. Iran. Med.* **2020**, *23*, 249–254. [CrossRef] [PubMed]
28. Cohen, J. *Statistical Power Analysis for the Behavioral Sciences*, 2nd ed.; Taylor & Francis: New York, NY, USA, 1988; p. 567.
29. Faul, F.; Erdfelder, E.; Buchner, A.; Lang, A.G. Statistical power analyses using G*Power 3.1: Tests for correlation and regression analyses. *Behav. Res. Methods* **2009**, *41*, 1149–1160. [CrossRef] [PubMed]
30. Ataş, O.; Talo Yildirim, T. Evaluation of knowledge, attitudes, and clinical education of dental students about COVID-19 pandemic. *PeerJ* **2020**, *8*, e9575. [CrossRef]
31. Harte, J.A. Standard and transmission-based precautions: An update for dentistry. *J. Am. Dent. Assoc.* **2010**, *141*, 572–581. [CrossRef] [PubMed]
32. Kohli, A.; Puttaiah, R. *Dental Infection Control and Occupational Safety for Oral Health Professionals*; Dental Council of India: New Delhi, India, 2008; p. 99.
33. Puttaiah, R.; Miller, K.; Bedi, D.R.; Shetty, S.; Almas, K.; Tse, E.; Kim, B.O.; Youngblood, D.; Minquan, D. Comparison of knowledge, attitudes and practice of dental safety from eight countries at the turn of the century. *J. Contemp. Dent. Pract.* **2011**, *12*, 1–7. [CrossRef] [PubMed]
34. World Health Organization. Effectiveness of Use of Chloroquine/Hydroxychloroquine in COVID-19 Case Management. 2020. Available online: https://www.afro.who.int/publications/effectiveness-use-chloroquine-hydroxychloroquine-covid-19-case-management (accessed on 12 October 2020).
35. Khader, Y.; Al Nsour, M.; Al-Batayneh, O.B.; Saadeh, R.; Bashier, H.; Alfaqih, M.; Al-Azzam, S.; AlShurman, B.A. Dentists' Awareness, Perception, and Attitude Regarding COVID-19 and Infection Control: Cross-Sectional Study Among Jordanian Dentists. *JMIR Public Health Surveill* **2020**, *6*, e18798. [CrossRef] [PubMed]
36. Singh, D.A. Knowledge, attitude and practice of medical and dental undergraduate students regarding COVID 19. *J. Med. Sci. Clin. Res.* **2020**, *08*, 645–652. [CrossRef]
37. Peng, Y.; Pei, C.; Zheng, Y.; Wang, J.; Zhang, K.; Zheng, Z.; Zhu, P. A cross-sectional survey of knowledge, attitude and practice associated with COVID-19 among undergraduate students in China. *BMC Public Health* **2020**, *20*, 1292. [CrossRef]
38. Iorfa, S.K.; Ottu, I.F.A.; Oguntayo, R.; Ayandele, O.; Olapegba, P.O. COVID-19 Knowledge, Risk Perception, and Precautionary Behavior Among Nigerians: A Moderated Mediation Approach. *Front Psychol.* **2020**, *11*, 566773. [CrossRef]

39. Davidson, D.J.; Freudenburg, W.R. Gender and environmental risk concerns. *Environ. Behav.* **1996**, *28*, 302–339. [CrossRef]
40. Kim, Y.; Park, I.; Kang, S. Age and gender differences in health risk perception. *Cent. Eur. J. Public Health* **2018**, *26*, 54–59. [CrossRef]
41. Maričić, J.; Sučić, I.; Šakić, V. Risk perception related to (Il)licit substance use and attitudes towards its' use and legalization–the role of age, gender and substance use. *Drus. Istraz.* **2013**, *22*, 579–599. [CrossRef]
42. Al-Hazmi, A.; Gosadi, I.; Somily, A.; Alsubaie, S.; Bin Saeed, A. Knowledge, attitude and practice of secondary schools and university students toward Middle East Respiratory Syndrome epidemic in Saudi Arabia: A cross-sectional study. *Saudi J. Biol. Sci.* **2018**, *25*, 572–577. [CrossRef] [PubMed]
43. Karaaslan, F.; Dikilitaş, A.; Aydin, E.Ö. Comparison of COVID-19 relevant knowledge and attitudes of clinical and preclinical dental students in Turkey. *Balk. J. Dent. Med.* **2020**, *24*, 1–7. [CrossRef]
44. Shahin, S.Y.; Bugshan, A.S.; Almulhim, K.S.; AlSharief, M.S.; Al-Dulaijan, Y.A.; Siddiqui, I.; al-Qarni, F.D. Knowledge of dentists, dental auxiliaries, and students regarding the COVID-19 pandemic in Saudi Arabia: A cross-sectional survey. *BMC Oral Health* **2020**, *20*, 363. [CrossRef] [PubMed]
45. Bennardo, F.; Buffone, C.; Fortunato, L.; Giudice, A. Are Dental Students Aware of and Knowledgeable about COVID-19? A Questionnaire-based Investigation. *Open Dent. J.* **2020**, *14*, 623–630. [CrossRef]
46. Almulhim, B.; Alasaaf, A.; Alghamdi, S.; Alroomy, R.; Aldhuwayhi, S.; Aljabr, A.; Mallineni, S.K. Dentistry Amidst the COVID-19 Pandemic: Knowledge, Attitude, and Practices Among the Saudi Arabian Dental Students. *Front. Med.* **2021**, *8*, 400. [CrossRef]
47. Ayub, A.; Goyal, A.; Kotwal, A.; Kulkarni, A.; Kotwal, A.; Mahen, A. Infection control practices in health care: Teaching and learning requirements of medical undergraduates. *Med. J. Armed Forces India* **2013**, *69*, 107–112. [CrossRef]
48. Varvara, G.; Bernardi, S.; Bianchi, S.; Sinjari, B.; Piattelli, M. Dental Education Challenges during the COVID-19 Pandemic Period in Italy: Undergraduate Student Feedback, Future Perspectives, and the Needs of Teaching Strategies for Professional Development. *Healthcare* **2021**, *9*, 454. [CrossRef]
49. Bianchi, S.; Gatto, R.; Fabiani, L. Effects of the SARS-COV-2 pandemic on medical education in Italy: Considerations and Tips. *Euro. Mediterr. Biomed. J.* **2020**, *15*, 100–102.
50. Bennardo, F.; Buffone, C.; Fortunato, L.; Giudice, A. COVID-19 is a challenge for dental education-A commentary. *Eur. J. Dent. Educ.* **2020**, *24*, 822–824. [CrossRef] [PubMed]

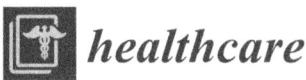

Article

Concerns, Knowledge, and Practices of Dentists in Mexico Regarding Infection Control during the Coronavirus Disease Pandemic: A Cross-Sectional Study

José F. Gómez-Clavel [1,*], Miguel A. Morales-Pérez [2], Gabriela Argumedo [3], Cynthia G. Trejo-Iriarte [4] and Alejandro García-Muñoz [4]

1. Laboratorio de Investigación en Educación y Odontología, Facultad de Estudios Superiores Iztacala, Universidad Nacional Autónoma de México, Tlalnepantla 54090, Mexico
2. Departamento de Cirugía Oral y Maxilofacial, Hospital Central Militar, Mexico City 11649, Mexico; miguel.amoralesperez@gmail.com
3. Departmento de Ciencias Experimentales, CCH Azcapotzalco, Universidad Nacional Autónoma de México, Azcapotzalco 02020, Mexico; cdargumedo@yahoo.com.mx
4. Laboratorio de Investigación Odontológica Almaraz, Facultad de Estudios Superiores Iztacala, Universidad Nacional Autónoma de México, Tlalnepantla 54090, Mexico; cynthia.belegii@gmail.com (C.G.T.-I.); alexondro_06@hotmail.com (A.G.-M.)
* Correspondence: gomclave@unam.mx; Tel.: +52-(553)-648-5058

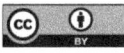

Citation: Gómez-Clavel, J.F.; Morales-Pérez, M.A.; Argumedo, G.; Trejo-Iriarte, C.G.; García-Muñoz, A. Concerns, Knowledge, and Practices of Dentists in Mexico Regarding Infection Control during the Coronavirus Disease Pandemic: A Cross-Sectional Study. *Healthcare* **2021**, *9*, 731. https://doi.org/10.3390/healthcare9060731

Academic Editors: Manoj Sharma and Kavita Batra

Received: 9 May 2021
Accepted: 12 June 2021
Published: 14 June 2021

Publisher's Note: MDPI stays neutral with regard to jurisdictional claims in published maps and institutional affiliations.

Copyright: © 2021 by the authors. Licensee MDPI, Basel, Switzerland. This article is an open access article distributed under the terms and conditions of the Creative Commons Attribution (CC BY) license (https://creativecommons.org/licenses/by/4.0/).

Abstract: Dentists are highly exposed and vulnerable during the coronavirus disease (COVID-19) pandemic, as physical proximity to patients is necessary for effective dental examination and treatment. The objective of this study was to describe the concerns, knowledge, and infection control practices of dentists in Mexico during the COVID-19 pandemic. In this cross-sectional study conducted from 22 May 2020 to 8 July 2020, an anonymous survey was distributed to dentists, which covered information regarding dentists' sociodemographic and professional characteristics, clinical practices during the pandemic, and perceptions regarding the application of infection prevention and control guidance for dental settings during the COVID-19 pandemic. Out of 703 respondents, 73.1% (*n* = 514) were women and 53.6% (*n* = 377) were dentists with 1–10 years of experience. Regarding the statements issued by the World Health Organization (WHO) and the Centers for Disease Control and Prevention (CDC), the responses for 11 survey items had total agreement rates >90% (high frequency); seven and nine items had moderate and low frequency of total agreement, respectively. Most dentists in this study agreed with the WHO and CDC statements and were concerned regarding the possibility of infection, despite using the protective gear.

Keywords: dentist; infection control practices; knowledge; concerns; COVID-19; SARS-CoV-2; pandemic; dental practice

1. Introduction

The spread of severe acute respiratory syndrome coronavirus 2 (SARS-CoV-2) virus has been established in most countries worldwide, including Mexico, and has led to the coronavirus disease (COVID-19) pandemic. This virus will possibly remain in our lives for a long time. It can be transmitted through direct, indirect, or close contact with the saliva, respiratory secretions, or respiratory droplets of infected persons. These droplets are usually >5–10 μm in diameter; droplets <5 μm in diameter are known as droplet nuclei or aerosols [1].

Effective prevention of oral health issues and optimal personal care remains a high priority during this COVID-19 pandemic [2]. Dentists are some of the most exposed and vulnerable healthcare professionals during this pandemic, mainly owing to the physical proximity that is necessary to effectively perform a dental examination on a patient [3]. In addition, the use of dental instruments usually generates aerosols, which can cause the air borne transmission of SARS-CoV-2 by remaining suspended in air over a long duration of time [4]. Therefore, each dental patient must be considered a possible carrier of the virus and maximum infection control measures should be applied to avoid viral transmission [3].

Dentists, as well as other health professionals, will have to continue their professional practice assuming that their everyday patients may have been infected with SARS-CoV-2, are asymptomatic, are in the incubation period and will subsequently develop symptoms, or are patients with COVID-19 infection.

In this current scenario, dentists must be able to provide adequate care by complying with the measures for infections control recommended by the World Health Organization (WHO) [2] and the Centers for Disease Control and Prevention (CDC) [5]. In Mexico, information on the number of dentists with dental practice, or verification of dentists' adherence to the recommended measures for infections prevention, is lacking. A study carried out in a small sample reported the changes made by Mexican dentists during the pandemic [6].

However, in this study, information related to the dentists' biosafety and economic concerns, their knowledge of protocols for infection control, and their sources of funding during the closure of their professional activity, is not addressed. Finally, we believe that the dentists' knowledge to prevent contagions during the pandemic is important information for the development of strategies that ensure that oral health professionals in Mexico are effectively informed and implement adequate security measures. Thus, the objective of this study was to describe the concerns, knowledge, and infection control practices of dentists in Mexico during the COVID-19 pandemic.

2. Materials and Methods

2.1. Study Design and Population

This was a cross-sectional study. An anonymous survey was designed, using Google's online survey system (Google Forms Questionnaire). The questionnaire consisted of 64 items categorized into three sections. The participating dentists were required to provide sociodemographic and professional information in Section 1. Information on the clinical practices of the participants during the COVID-19 pandemic was required in Section 2. The perception of the dentists on the application of the 'Interim Infection Prevention and Control Guidance for Dental Settings During the COVID-19 Pandemic' was explored in Section 3, using a Likert scale [2,4]. The questionnaire was distributed through the social networks of different dental associations between 22 May 2020 and 18 July 2020. Paramedical staff and dental students were not included in this survey.

The Ethics Committee of the Faculty of Higher Studies, Iztacala, at the National Autonomous University of Mexico granted ethical approval for this study and for the use of survey results and responses (CE/FESI/062020/1357). Informed consent to participate in the study was obtained from all participants. This study and its methods followed all relevant guidelines and regulations, in accordance with the Declaration of Helsinki.

2.2. Sample Size Calculation

The required sample size was 707, with an "n" of the study universe of 100,000, a heterogeneity of 50%, a margin of error of 2%, and a confidence level of 95%. The sample size was calculated by using the online Netquest calculator (https://www.netquest.com/es/calculadora-tamano-muestra; accessed on 20 May 2020). The response acceptance was closed (18 July 2020) when the required sample size was nearly achieved and there were no new responses for 10 days.

2.3. Statistical Analysis

The data were statistically analyzed using SPSS version 21.0 for Windows (IBM Corp., Armonk, NY, USA). Descriptive statistics (frequencies and percentages) were used to describe the quantitative and categorical variables. The Mann–Whitney and Kruskal–

Wallis tests were used to assess differences in mean values for Likert scale items. The level of significance was set at $p < 0.05$.

3. Results

A total of 703 dental surgeons completed the survey; 73% of the respondents were women. Regarding the participants' experience in dental practice, 54%, 21%, 13%, and 12.7% of the respondents had 1–10, 11–20, 21–30, and ≥31 years of experience, respectively. Regarding the type of dental practice, 6% of the respondents practiced in a government institution, 51% owned their clinic, 24% worked on contract in a private clinic, 19% underwent both institutional and private practice, and 45% of the participants were general practice dentists (Table 1).

Table 1. Sociodemographic characteristics of the participants.

Variables	$n = 703$	%
Sex		
Female	514	73
Male	189	27
Years of clinical experience		
1–10	377	54
11–20	145	21
21–30	92	13
>30	89	12.7
Type of dental practice		
Institutional	44	6.3
Private, I am the owner	356	51
Private, I am not the owner	170	24
Institutional and private	133	19
Specialty		
General practice (not specialist)	321	45
Orthodontics	210	30
Endodontics	48	6.8
Pediatric dentistry	28	4
Other types of postgraduate degree	26	3.7
Prosthetics/rehabilitation	23	3.3
Periodontics	22	3.1
Oral/maxillofacial Surgery	20	2.8
Pathology	5	0.7

Out of the 703 respondents, 197 stated that they worked during the national program of the Mexican Ministry of Health called "Jornada Nacional de Sana Distancia" (National Journey of Healthy Distance). The program was implemented with an aim to contain the COVID-19 pandemic in Mexico, and it was conducted between 23 March 2020 and 30 May 2020. Among dentists who reported that they closed their clinic, 197 closed their offices during March–June (134 in March, 48 in April, 7 in May, and 3 in June); 171 closed their offices following the recommendations of the Mexican Ministry of Health; and one reported that he was infected and developed COVID-19. Among the respondents who did not have a dental practice, 31% overcame their lack of income by managing their savings, 22% earned income from other activities not related to dentistry, and 18% received financial assistance from their families. The activities performed by the dentists who stayed at home were mainly hobbies ($n = 73$), exercise ($n = 47$), and spending time with family ($n = 47$); only 21 (11%) reported that they conducted classes or attended dental lectures online (Table 2).

Table 2. Activities of dentists who did not work during the active phase of the pandemic.

	n = 197	%
Date of office closure or halting work		
March	134	68
April	48	24.4
May	7	3.6
June	3	1.5
Did not respond	5	2.53
Dental office was closed because:		
I followed the general recommendations for the control of the pandemic	171	86.8
I found out that a colleague was infected	1	0.5
Someone close to me was infected (friend or relative)	5	2.5
No patient wanted to attend a consultation	4	2
Some third party forced me (my boss, landlord, partner, others)	2	1
I got COVID-19	1	0.5
Did not respond	13	6.6
Source of income (n = 197)		
I received income from a private clinic/office	10	5
I received income from a public clinic/clinic	11	5.6
I received income from another job not related to dentistry	44	22.3
I received financial support from a government agency	6	3
I received financial support from close family/friends	35	17.8
I managed with my savings	60	30.5
I received loans or credit (institutional, bank)	5	2.5
I received income as a teacher	21	1.5
Did not respond	5	2.5
I dedicated my free time at home to (n = 197):		
Hobbies (guitar, drawing, music, cooking, others)	73	37
Exercise/Sports	47	24
Family	47	24
Online dentistry classes, courses, or conferences	21	11
Studying or reading on my own	5	3
Watching television, series, movies	1	0.5
Did not respond	3	1.5

Among the 506 dentists who reported that they worked between April and June, only 14% stated that they worked under the normal conditions, while the remaining 86% worked under different conditions. Among the 436 dentists who worked under different conditions, only 60% attended to emergencies and 26% attended to patients who were undergoing previously initiated treatments. In total, 444 dentists performed high-risk dental activities; 73% used a dental air water spray and 80% used a handpiece. The dental procedures performed by dentists who were working during the active phase of the pandemic were as follows: dental examination and prescription of non-steroidal anti-inflammatory drugs (NSAIDs) and antibiotics (69.4%), exodontia (63%), diagnosis (59%), and endodontics (46%) (Table 3).

The infection transmission control measures applied before consultation were frequent cleaning of surfaces in between consultations (97%), asking patients to rub their hands with alcohol gel (90%), and placement of disinfectant mats with 0.5% sodium hypochlorite in the clinic (70%). The personal protective equipment (PPE) that the dentists used included heat-sealed, three-layer surgical masks (47%), N95 respirators (60.3%), gloves (98%), and face shields (94%). The agents used to disinfect the surfaces of the office prior to the consultation included sodium hypochlorite solution (58%), Lysol (54%), disinfectant wipes (47%), alcohol (23.7%), and liquid detergents (17%) (Table 4).

Table 3. Work patterns of dentists who worked during the active phase of the pandemic.

	n = 506	%
I worked normally	70	14
To complete unfinished treatments	131	25.9
I only attended to emergencies	305	60.2
I turned on the air compressor	444	87.7
I used dental air water spray triple syringe	367	73
I used dental handpiece	406	80.2
Type of treatments performed during the pandemic(one alternative do not exclude others)	F	%
Dental examination and prescription of NSAIDs and antibiotics	351	69.4
Exodontia	320	63.2
Diagnosis	300	59.2
Endodontics	232	45.8
Operative dentistry	208	41.1
Pathology	190	37.5
Dental prosthesis	130	25.7
Periodontics	64	12.6
Orthodontics	64	12.6

NSAIDs, non-steroidal anti-inflammatory drugs

Table 4. Prevention of transmission during clinical dental care (multiple selections possible).

	n = 506	%
Control measures performed prior to dental care:		
Placement of disinfectant mats with sodium hypochlorite concentrations of at least 0.5% in the clinic	355	70
Request that patients wash their hands	324	90
Request patients to rub their hands with alcohol gel	453	90
Administer a questionnaire to inquire about the places the patient visited and explore respiratory symptoms	310	61.2
Measurement of temperature	304	60
Request patients rinse hands with chlorhexidine or hydrogen peroxide	341	67.4
Frequent cleaning of surfaces in between consultations	488	96.5
PPE used		
Goggles	367	73
Face shield mask	476	94
Simple two-layer surgical mask	119	24
Heat-sealed three-layer surgical mask	239	47.2
N95 respirator or equivalent	305	60.3
PPE overalls	223	44
Surgical cap	437	86.4
Gloves	498	98.4
Disposable surgical boots	164	32.4
Substances used to disinfect surfaces before care interventions		
Lysol	275	54.3
Chlorine	291	58
Alcohol	120	23.7
Liquid detergent	88	17.4
Disinfectant wipes	238	47

PPE, personal protective equipment.

The percentages, by which these measures increased the costs of services by 10%, 20%, and 30%, were 19%, 8%, and 3%, respectively. The main reasons some dentists did not increase the costs of dental services included solidarity with patients (41%), the fact that the budgets were previously agreed upon (15%), or because they had reserve materials (10%).

Among the dentists who worked, 61% indicated that the number of patients they saw per day was 1–3, 68% (n = 344) reported that they did not increase the costs of their services, and 32% increased them. Those who increased the cost of their services reported that the increase was mainly attributed to the increase in the cost of inputs (26%) and the use of more PPE (4.2%). Regarding teleconsultation, 186 dentists reported that they did not provide remote consultation. Among those who provided remote consultation, most used WhatsApp (n = 290), telephone calls (n = 214), and video conferencing (n = 55) (Table 5).

Table 5. Accounting in the office.

	F	%	n = 506
Average number of patients seen			
1–3	309	61	
4–7	132	26	
>7	47	9.3	
They did not respond	18	3.6	
Increased the costs of their services	162	32	
Reasons for increasing costs			
Increased cost of materials and equipment	132	26	
Use of more PPE	21	4.2	
Because of the risk we run during the pandemic	5	1	
Percentage of dental services cost increase			
10%	95	18.8	
20%	39	7.7	
30%	20	3.4	
40%	5	1	
Reasons for not increasing costs			
The budgets had been agreed in advance	77	15.2	
I had reserve material	51	10	
Out of solidarity with my patients and my country	209	41.3	
Media used for remote consultation (multiple response)			
Phone call	214	42.3	
Email	14	2.8	
WhatsApp	290	57.3	
Videoconference (Google Meet, Zoom)	55	10.9	
Social Networks (i.e., Facebook, Twitter, Blog)	40	7.9	
Messages (SMS)	35	6.9	
I do not give remote consultation	186	36.8	

PPE, personal protective equipment.

The perception of the dentists regarding the recommendations or statements on biosecurity in the dental clinic issued by different organizations was also measured.

Regarding general knowledge on working safely during the COVID-19 pandemic, the statement that had the highest frequency of total agreement was item 34 ("the virus that causes COVID-19 is spread primarily through respiratory drops when an infected person coughs, sneezes, or speaks"); 11 items had a percentage of total agreement > 90%, seven and nine items had a moderate and a low frequency of total agreement, respectively (Table 6).

Regarding the concerns of dentists concerning the effectiveness of preventive measures against the transmission of SARS-CoV-2, 88.5% agreed with statement 38 ("face masks do not provide complete protection against inhalation of airborne infectious agents such as SARS-CoV-2"), 86.5% agreed with statement 47 ("I am concerned that I may become infected despite using PPE"), and 88% agreed with statement 59 ("I will continue with the same measures that I have worked with during the pandemic"). These statements had the highest frequencies of agreement. In addition, the dentists were concerned regarding the economic impact of the pandemic on their clinics. Details of the economic concerns, the perception of the dentists regarding the characteristics of dental settings, and how they see the future, are summarized in Table 7.

Table 6. General knowledge of the dentists regarding working safely during the COVID-19 pandemic (n = 703).

Statement	Agree with the Statement (%)	Source of Statement
The virus that causes COVID-19 is spread primarily through respiratory drops when an infected person coughs, sneezes, or speaks.	97.7	CDC-WHO
Dentists and their assistants should be considered professionals at high exposure risk, as their practice has a high potential for exposure to known or suspected sources of the virus that causes COVID-19 during specific procedures.	97.2	WHO
It is important not to use a cellphone while caring for my patients.	97	CDC
Asymptomatic individuals or those in the incubation period may also be able to transmit SARS-CoV-2.	96.7	CDC-
During dental procedures, the use of the handpiece or ultrasonic scaler and the triple syringe produce a visible aerosol containing large droplets of water particles, saliva, blood, microorganisms, and other debris.	96.7	WHO
I must consider that every patient who comes to the office is potentially a transmitter of SARS-CoV-2.	96.2	CDC
I must proactively communicate to staff and patients the need to stay home if they are ill.	95	CDC
Dentists are directly exposed to inhalation of viral particles in aerosols, where the virus can remain viable for up to 3 h.	93.6	WHO
It is important for the office to have good natural ventilation.	93.6	CDC-WHO
If a patient comes to the office and is suspected or confirmed to have COVID-19, I should defer dental treatment.	92.7	CDC
Aerosols generated by using a dental handpiece or dental air water spray travel a short distance and land on the floor and surfaces of the dental unit and on the patient.	91.5	WHO
I must record everyone's temperature before they enter the office.	88.5	CDC
The virus survives in aerosols for hours and on some surfaces for days.	88.8	WHO
During the COVID-19 pandemic, the dental clinic or office has unique characteristics that warrant additional considerations for infection control.	85.3	CDC
It is necessary to verify that my N95 respirator has been approved by the NIOSH.	84.8	CDC
Using the rubber dam can minimize the production of aerosols contaminated with saliva and blood when I use the high-speed handpiece.	84.6	WHO
To ensure that infection control is up to high quality standards, the dental procedures must be done in an infection isolation room.	82.1	CDC
During and after the COVID-19 pandemic, the use of N95 respirators becomes necessary.	80.4	CDC-WHO
During the pandemic, I must postpone elective procedures, surgeries, and non-urgent reviews or consultations in the clinic.	78.2	CDC-WHO
Disinfection of the patient's footwear is useful. [1]	74.3	
It is important that the patient use a mouthwash with 1% hydrogen.	67.7	CDC
To inactivate SARS-CoV-2 in the handpiece, I have to use heat sterilization.	66.4	CDC
It is important to work with an assistant.	58.7	WHO
I can work alone without an assistant.	48.6	WHO
It is useful to use a rinse with chlorhexidine to inactivate the SARS-CoV-2 present in the mucosa and saliva.	47.4	WHO
To inactivate SARS-CoV-2 in the handpiece, simply immerse it in a 70% alcohol solution for 15 min.	33.7	CDC
It is important that the office has air conditioning.	17.8	CDC-WHO

[1] Local guideline. COVID-19, coronavirus disease; CDC, Centers for Disease Control and Prevention; WHO, World Health Organization; NIOSH, National Institute for Occupational Safety and Health; SARS-CoV-2, severe acute respiratory syndrome coronavirus 2. There were no differences based on sex (Mann–Whitney, $p > 0.05$) or years of experience (Kruskal–Wallis, $p > 0.05$) for any of the items.

Table 7. Concerns regarding the COVID-19 pandemic and the effectiveness of preventive measures against its transmission.

Item	Statement	Agree with the Statement (%)	Mean	SD
38	Face mask does not provide complete protection against inhalation of airborne infectious agents, such as SARS-CoV-2.	88.5	4.3	0.9
59	I will continue with the same measures that I worked with during the pandemic.	88	3.8	1.2
47	I am concerned that I may become infected despite using PPE.	86.5	3.8	1.1
39	No data to assess the risk of transmission during dental treatment.	70	4.3	0.9
54	Surgical masks or face masks are not designed to protect the user from inhaling viral particles.	70	3.8	1
51	Standard protective measures in daily clinical practice are not effective enough to prevent the transmission of SARS-CoV-2.	70	1.8	0.9
60	It will no longer be necessary to have as many preventive measures.	4.6	4.3	0.9
	Concerns regarding the economic impact of COVID-19 pandemic			
62	The costs of implementing measures to ensure stricter protection barriers will increase the costs of my services.	88.8	4.1	0.9
61	I believe the economic impact on my office will be severe.	77.4	4.1	0.9

There were no differences in responses based on sex (Mann–Whitney, $p > 0.05$) or years of experience (Kruskal–Wallis, $p > 0.05$) for any of the items. COVID-19, coronavirus disease; SARS-CoV-2, severe acute respiratory syndrome coronavirus 2; SD, standard deviation; PPE, personal protective equipment.

4. Discussion

In this study, we aimed to describe the attitude, knowledge, and infection control practices of dentists in Mexico during the COVID-19 pandemic. Although it is still too early to be certain regarding the general trends of the clinical experiences of dentists on the transmission of COVID-19 during dental care, this study outlines their perceptions, attitudes, and concerns during the pandemic. Most of the dentists performed risky procedures, such as turning on air compressors and using handpieces. The use of the dental handpiece and triple syringe are considered biological risk factors in the transmission of COVID-19, as they favor the diffusion of aerosol particles from saliva, blood, and secretions [7,8]. In addition, since SARS-CoV-2 can persist in aerosols for up to 3 h and has a relatively long half-life of approximately 1.1–1.2 h, this aerosol production facilitates the contamination of the environment, including the dental surfaces, instruments, and appliances [9]. The most frequent activity performed in the clinic was patient screening and the prescription of antibiotics and NSAIDs, which probably led to an increase in the prescription of antibiotics during the months of the pandemic, as reported by an English team [10].

Regarding the general knowledge of dentists on working safely during the COVID-19 pandemic, most respondents indirectly showed good knowledge of concepts and attitudes as demonstrated through their degree of agreement to work according to the guidelines obtained from the scientific literature and the provisional guidelines of the CDC [5] and the WHO [2].

Our survey showed that 72% of the respondents worked during the active phase of the pandemic, a percentage that is similar to that reported for Brazilian dentists (64%) [11]. The main types of treatments performed by dentists in Mexico were related to dental pain, in line with the results of the previous work [11]. Since the start of the pandemic, teleconsultation has become an auxiliary mean of delivering dental services related to education, consultation, and triage [12]. The medium most frequently used for teleconsultation among dentists in our study was WhatsApp (58%), whereas in the study performed in Brazil, the frequency of its use was up to 70.6% [11].

Our results were similar to those reported by Kamate et al. [13], Nasser et al. [14], and Sesgin et al. [15]. These studies also reported that dentists had good knowledge and practice scores, which are important in the prevention of COVID-19. They advised dentists to follow the guidelines of the CDC [5] and the WHO [2] in their clinics, and to sensitize their staff on the best biosecurity practices to ensure that the effects of this pandemic are mitigated.

However, responses to certain items in the questionnaire reflect practices that are not in full accordance with the recommended guidelines for infection control as established in the Guidelines for Infection Control in Dental Health-Care Settings [16]. For example, regarding the guideline for heat sterilization of the dental handpiece, only 66.4% of the respondents agreed, whereas 33.7% agreed with the following statement: "To inactivate SARS-CoV-2 in the handpiece, simply immerse it in a 70% alcohol solution for 15 min." This practice is specifically flagged as an unacceptable and unsafe sterilization method [16,17].

Another risky practice is not following the WHO recommendation when using the handpiece, which is working with four hands; only 58.7% agreed that it is important to work with an assistant, whereas 77% indicated that they can work without an assistant. In addition, regarding working with a rubber dam and using a respirator, such as N95 or FFP2, 80.4% and 84.6% agreed with the use of N95 respirators and rubber dam, respectively; both results were consistent with those reported in another survey conducted in Mexico [6]. The use of the rubber dam has traditionally been looked down on, even among endodontists [18]. However, given the risk of generating aerosols during clinical dental work, the importance of its use among general practice dentists has to be reconsidered [19,20]. Another critical point in the work of dentists is in relation to the ventilation requirements that the operating room must have. The current recommendation is that it must be well ventilated or have an air conditioning system with EPA filters [2,21].

In a survey conducted in Poland, 71.2% of the dentists who responded to the questionnaire decided to suspend clinical practice during that specific reported time [22]. In our study population, only 28% stopped working during the study period, in contrary to the results reported by Casillas et al., which stated that only 14.8% did not attend to patients [6]. Perhaps the dentists in Mexico worked during the study period because of financial need or because they are used to following infection control protocols as established in the Guidelines for Infection Control in Dental Health-Care Settings, thus, making them confident enough to work during that period [16]. In the Polish survey, the authors reported that the main factor behind the decision to suspend clinical practice was the shortage of PPE, unlike the present study in which the participants reported that the application of the general recommendations for pandemic control was the main cause of work suspension in the office. Some elements of our survey explore the concerns of dentists, which was mainly that, despite protective measures, they may become infected. The dentists in the Polish study expressed a general feeling of anxiety and uncertainty regarding the COVID-19 situation. Another study indicated that despite having a high level of knowledge and practice, dentists worldwide are in a state of anxiety and fear while working in their respective fields [23].

Knowledge of infection control practices in the dental community may enable the reaffirmation of professional training recommendations and may serve to update the programs of dental curriculums at the undergraduate and postgraduate levels as well as in continuing education courses. This would allow dentists to become aware of the possible mistakes that may occur in professional practice and would allow for the provision of a safe clinical environment for the benefit of dentists and patients.

At the time of the survey, only one dentist claimed to have been infected with SARS-CoV-2. However, as dental office care routines are activated, more dentists are likely to be affected by COVID-19, because they were infected in their dental practice or through other activities.

Regarding concerns about the efficacy of preventive measures for SARS-CoV-2, the face mask mentioned in item 38 does not provide complete protection against the inhalation of airborne infectious agents. Ideally, the transmission of SARS-CoV-2 among dentists should be monitored. We hope that the arrival of a vaccine will allow dentists to work without fear. However, this can be done only with the awareness of maximizing the use of protective barriers to avoid the transmission of infectious diseases and applying prevention protocols against the spread of COVID-19 [24]. Although the data collection was conducted within a 2 month period, it is well known that multiple revisions on the guidelines for the management of COVID-19 have been recommended from the initial stages of the pandemic by organizations, such as the CDC. These modified recommendations do not always reach the dental professionals promptly. Therefore, it is essential to monitor these changes and promote their dissemination.

The limitations of this study should be noted. As this was a cross-sectional study and the survey was conducted online, the risk of bias cannot be ruled out. In addition, no sampling technique was used to make the study representative. Therefore, the results of this survey cannot be generalized.

5. Conclusions

In conclusion, most of the surveyed dentists worked during the pandemic. They had a good level of knowledge regarding the transmission routes of SARS-CoV-2 and infection control measures to manage and care for patients and themselves. However, there are great concerns regarding the possibility of becoming infected and suffering from COVID-19.

Author Contributions: Conceptualization, J.F.G.-C. and G.A.; methodology, J.F.G.-C., G.A., M.A.M.-P. and A.G.; formal analysis, J.F.G.-C. and C.T.; investigation, J.F.G.-C. and C.G.T.-I.; writing—original draft preparation, J.F.G.-C., G.A. and A.G.-M.; writing—review and editing, J.F.G.-C., M.A.M.-P., G.A., C.G.T.-I. and A.G.-M. All authors have read and agreed to the published version of the manuscript.

Funding: This research received no external funding.

Institutional Review Board Statement: The study was conducted according to the guidelines of the Declaration of Helsinki and approved by the Ethics Committee of the Faculty of Higher Studies, Iztacala, (FES) at the UNAM (CE/FESI/062020/1357).

Informed Consent Statement: Written informed consent was obtained from all subjects involved in the study.

Data Availability Statement: The datasets used and/or analyzed during the current study are available from the corresponding author on reasonable request.

Conflicts of Interest: The authors declare no conflict of interest.

References

1. Fennelly, K.P. Particle sizes of infectious aerosols: Implications for infection control. *Lancet Respir. Med.* **2020**, *8*, 914–924. [CrossRef]
2. Considerations for the Provision of Essential Oral Health Services in the Context of COVID-19: Interim Guidance, 3 August 2020. World Health Organization. Available online: https://apps.who.int/iris/handle/10665/333625 (accessed on 14 August 2020).
3. Which Occupations Have the Highest Potential Exposure to the Coronavirus (COVID-19)? Office for National Statistics. Available online: https://www.ons.gov.uk/employmentandlabourmarket/peopleinwork/employmentandemployeetypes/articles/whichoccupationshavethehighestpotentialexposuretothecoronaviruscovid19/2020-05-11 (accessed on 6 October 2020).
4. Transmission of SARSCoV-2: Implications for Infection Prevention Precautions: Scientific Brief, 09 July 2020. World Health Organization. Available online: https://apps.who.int/iris/handle/10665/333114 (accessed on 14 August 2020).
5. Interim Infection Prevention and Control Guidance for Dental Settings during the COVID-19 Response. Centers for Disease Control and Prevention. Available online: https://www.cdc.gov/coronavirus/2019-ncov/hcp/dental-settings.html (accessed on 8 April 2020).
6. Casillas Santana, M.Á.; Martínez Zumarán, A.; Patiño Marín, N.; Castillo Silva, B.E.; Sámano Valencia, C.; Salas Orozco, M.F. How dentists face the COVID-19 in Mexico: A nationwide cross-sectional study. *Int. J. Environ. Res. Public Health* **2021**, *18*, 1750. [CrossRef] [PubMed]
7. Ge, Z.Y.; Yang, L.M.; Xia, J.J.; Fu, X.H.; Zhang, Y.Z. Possible aerosol transmission of COVID-19 and special precautions in dentistry. *J. Zhejiang Univ. Sci. B.* **2020**, *21*, 361–368. [CrossRef] [PubMed]
8. Peng, X.; Xu, X.; Li, Y.; Cheng, L.; Zhou, X.; Ren, B. Transmission routes of 2019-nCoV and controls in dental practice. *Int. J. Oral Sci.* **2020**, *12*, 9. [CrossRef] [PubMed]
9. van Doremalen, N.; Bushmaker, T.; Morris, D.H.; Holbrook, M.G.; Gamble, A.; Williamson, B.N.; Tamin, D.H.; Harcourt, J.L.; Thornburg, N.J.; Gerber, S.I.; et al. Aerosol and surface stability of SARS-CoV-2 as compared with SARS-CoV-1. *N. Engl. J. Med.* **2020**, *382*, 1564–1567. [CrossRef] [PubMed]
10. Wordley, V.; Shah, S.; Thompson, W. Increased antibiotics use. *Br. Dent. J.* **2020**, *229*, 266. [CrossRef] [PubMed]

11. Faccini, M.; Ferruzzi, F.; Mori, A.A.; Santin, G.C.; Oliveira, R.C.; Oliveira, R.C.G.; Queiroz, P.M.; Salmeron, S.; Pini, N.I.P.; Sunfeld, D.; et al. Dental care during COVID-19 outbreak: A web-based survey. *Eur. J. Dent.* **2020**, *14*, S14–S19. [CrossRef] [PubMed]
12. Brian, Z.; Weintraub, J.A. Oral health and COVID-19: Increasing the need for prevention and access. *Prev. Chronic Dis.* **2020**, *17*, E82. [CrossRef] [PubMed]
13. Kamate, S.K.; Sharma, S.; Thakar, S.; Srivastava, D.; Sengupta, K.; Hadi, A.J.; Chaudhary, A.; Joshi, R.; Dhanker, K. Assessing knowledge, attitudes and practices of dental practitioners regarding the COVID-19 pandemic: A multinational study. *Dent. Med. Probl.* **2020**, *57*, 11–17. [CrossRef] [PubMed]
14. Nasser, Z.; Fares, Y.; Daoud, R.; Abou-Abbas, L. Assessment of knowledge and practice of dentists towards coronavirus disease (COVID-19): A cross-sectional survey from Lebanon. *BMC Oral Health* **2020**, *20*, 281. [CrossRef] [PubMed]
15. Sezgin, G.P.; ŞirinoĞlu Çapan, B. Assessment of dentists' awareness and knowledge levels on the Novel Coronavirus (COVID-19). *Braz. Oral Res.* **2020**, *34*, e112. [CrossRef] [PubMed]
16. Kohn, W.G.; Collins, A.S.; Cleveland, J.L.; Harte, J.A.; Eklund, K.J.; Malvitz, D.M. Guidelines for infection control in dental health-care settings–2003. *MMWR Recomm. Rep.* **2003**, *52*, 1–61. [CrossRef] [PubMed]
17. Pinto, F.M.; Bruna, C.Q.; Camargo, T.C.; Marques, M.; Silva, C.B.; Sasagawa, S.M.; Mimica, L.M.J.; Graziano, K.U. The practice of disinfection of high-speed handpieces with 70% w/v alcohol: An evaluation. *Am. J. Infect. Control* **2017**, *45*, e19–e22. [CrossRef] [PubMed]
18. Madarati, A.A. Why dentists don't use rubber dam during endodontics and how to promote its usage? *BMC Oral Health* **2016**, *16*, 24. [CrossRef] [PubMed]
19. Hill, E.E.; Rubel, B.S. Do dental educators need to improve their approach to teaching rubber dam use? *J. Dent. Educ.* **2008**, *72*, 1177–1181. [CrossRef] [PubMed]
20. Villani, F.A.; Aiuto, R.; Paglia, L.; Re, D. COVID-19 and dentistry: Prevention in dental practice, a literature review. *Int. J. Environ. Res. Public Health* **2020**, *17*, 4609. [CrossRef] [PubMed]
21. Ashtiani, R.E.; Tehrani, S.; Revilla-León, M.; Zandinejad, A. Reducing the risk of COVID-19 transmission in dental offices: A review. *J. Prosthodont.* **2020**, *20*, 275. [CrossRef] [PubMed]
22. Tysiąc-Miśta, M.; Dziedzic, A. The attitudes and professional approaches of dental practitioners during the COVID-19 outbreak in Poland: A cross-sectional survey. *Int. J. Environ. Res. Public Health* **2020**, *17*, 4703. [CrossRef] [PubMed]
23. Ahmed, M.A.; Jouhar, R.; Ahmed, N.; Adnan, S.; Aftab, M.; Zafar, M.S.; Khurshid, Z. Fear and practice modifications among dentists to combat novel Coronavirus Disease (COVID-19) outbreak. *Int. J. Environ. Res. Public Health* **2020**, *17*, 2821. [CrossRef] [PubMed]
24. Amato, A.; Caggiano, M.; Amato, M.; Moccia, G.; Capunzo, M.; De Caro, F. Infection control in dental practice during the COVID-19 pandemic. *Int. J. Environ. Res. Public Health* **2020**, *17*, 4769. [CrossRef] [PubMed]

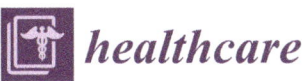

Article

Assessment of Awareness and Knowledge on Novel Coronavirus (COVID-19) Pandemic among Seafarers

Gopi Battineni [1,*], Getu Gamo Sagaro [1], Nalini Chintalapudi [1], Marzio Di Canio [2] and Francesco Amenta [1,2]

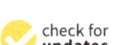

- [1] Telemedicine and Telepharmacy Centre, School of Medicinal and Health Products Sciences, University of Camerino, 62032 Camerino, Italy; getugamo.sagaro@unicam.it (G.G.S.); nalini.chintalapudi@unicam.it (N.C.); francesco.amenta@unicam.it (F.A.)
- [2] Research Department, Centro Internationale Radio Medico (C.I.R.M), 00144 Rome, Italy; mdicanio@cirmservizi.it
- * Correspondence: gopi.battineni@unicam.it; Tel.: +39-3331728206

Citation: Battineni, G.; Sagaro, G.G.; Chintalapudi, N.; Di Canio, M.; Amenta, F. Assessment of Awareness and Knowledge on Novel Coronavirus (COVID-19) Pandemic among Seafarers. *Healthcare* **2021**, *9*, 120. https://doi.org/10.3390/healthcare9020120

Academic Editors: Manoj Sharma, Kavita Batra and Tao-Hsin Tung
Received: 21 December 2020
Accepted: 19 January 2021
Published: 25 January 2021

Publisher's Note: MDPI stays neutral with regard to jurisdictional claims in published maps and institutional affiliations.

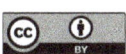

Copyright: © 2021 by the authors. Licensee MDPI, Basel, Switzerland. This article is an open access article distributed under the terms and conditions of the Creative Commons Attribution (CC BY) license (https://creativecommons.org/licenses/by/4.0/).

Abstract: *Background*: The ongoing pandemic due to the novel coronavirus (COVID-19) is becoming a serious global threat. Experts suggest that the infection can be controlled by immediate prevention measures. Sailing is one of the occupational categories more vulnerable to this virus outbreak due to the proximity of the working conditions. *Objective*: Awareness and knowledge assessments of seafarers towards the current epidemic is mandatory to understand the effectiveness and success of the infection control measures adopted by shipping companies. *Methods:* In this study, we presented an online questionnaire survey to determine the knowledge levels of COVID-19 among seafarers. The data were collected by self-reported survey, and analysis was done by the analysis of variance (ANOVA). The *t*-test was used to understand the knowledge attitude differences to COVID-19 among different occupational groups of seafarers, and the *p*-value $\leq$ of 0.05 was considered statistically significant. *Results:* Among 1,458 responses received, 92.82% had a college or university degree. The results reported that the mean COVID-19 knowledge score was 5.82 (standard deviation = 0.51, range 0–6), and the overall correct percentage was 97%. There was a statistically significant difference between age groups (F (4, 1453) = 5.44, $p < 0.001$) and educational groups (F (4, 1453) = 1.52, $p < 0.001$). The knowledge score was not significantly different across the educational status of the participants (F (2, 1455) = 1.52, $p = 0.220$). *Conclusions*: The present study highlighted good knowledge and behaviours among sailors about COVID-19. However, shipping companies need to come up with new campaigns to hold optimistic practices and suitable guidelines on ships, including cruise boats, to keep sea workers always alert and collaborative in mitigating the spread of COVID-19.

Keywords: COVID-19 spreading; online survey; awareness and knowledge; ships; seafarers

1. Introduction

The novel coronavirus disease, or COVID-19, was first identified in December 2019 at a Wuhan wet market in China and then constantly spread all over the world at a rapid pace [1]. As of 5 January 2021, more than 85 million cases have been reported, including 1.86 million deaths [2]. In many cases, COVID-19 develops mild-to-moderate symptoms. In some cases, it might cause severe sickness, including pneumonia and, consequently, death. A person who is infected by the virus usually takes five to seven days to develop symptoms, and it can extend up to 14 days [3].

Currently, many European countries like Italy, France, Germany, and others have been exposed to the second wave of the COVID-19 pandemic [4]. These countries were severely hit by the first wave of pandemic during the spring, which was followed by the second wave during late summer and autumn. Epidemic data present the virus characteristics, and its effects are varied between these two periods. The symptoms like pneumonia, dyspnea, fever, cough, chronic neurological diseases, and type 2 diabetes mellitus are often found in both waves. In severe cases, the symptoms usually get worse gradually after the initial appearance. To slow down the spreading of the virus and reduce its effects, governments around the world have made travel restrictions and closed their country's borders [5]. Various ports and air terminals are closed, ships' entries are denied, and all planes grounded.

Due to the limited medical resources, natural exposure to new environments and crowded, enclosed areas make the high risk of the present novel pandemic spread among many cruise ships [6]. On 4 February 2020, the UK-registered ship named the Diamond Princess was exposed to a large outbreak of COVID-19, and this was quarantined for about one month at Yokohama, Japan. More than 700 individuals were infected, including 14 deaths [7]. Over 40 cruise ships have confirmed positive cases of COVID-19 infection onboard, and port authorities and governments are advising people to avoid travelling on cruise ships and restraining ships from docking [8]. Besides, many maritime transport lines have been suspended to prevent the epidemic spread [9].

Seafarers are the unsung heroes of this pandemic, because over 90% of the world trade, including medical goods, raw materials, essential foods, and manufactured goods, depends on them [10]. Based on a report published by the International Maritime Organization (IMO), seafarers are collateral victims of this pandemic emergency, as travel limitations have left a huge number of them abandoned on boats or unfit to join ships [11]. Moreover, commercial fishing is a main source of the world's food. Several sailors are ready for stretched out work timeframes; to maintain a strategic distance from becoming infected, crewmembers need to change all the time, and this includes nearly 100,000 sailors every month [12,13].

The COVID-19 pandemic has introduced phenomenal circumstances around the world. The worldwide health authorities have been focused on controlling the disease by mitigating actions to limit the fast-spreading. Currently, two vaccines—namely, Pfizer-BioNtech and Moderna's—are authorized and recommended to prevent COVID-19; additionally, the presence of more than 50 COVID-19 vaccines are in trials, yet the world is looking for safe and effective ones [14]. Of the problems caused by the COVID-19 pandemic, around 90,000 sailors are now stuck on cruise ships without passengers [15]. Since the ship is a closed environment, there is a high chance of being infected. After being at sea for at least 14 days, and if no crewmember shows the symptoms of the COVID-19 illness, then a ship can be considered as virus-free and, eventually, safe.

The recent literature on COVID-19 highlights scientific knowledge or epidemic projections, especially in the public health environment [16]. Outcomes integrated with scientific knowledge tend to identify the key safety-related issues. Apart from the clinical and healthcare aspects like the safety of medical doctors, social and occupational safety, and, in particular, mental health, they have gained large attention from the COVID-19 scientific community [17]. The individuals living in closed environments like ships should have basic knowledge when addressing key social issues, including an urgent need to understand and believe the science about the COVID-19 pandemic that is shattering the present world.

This study presents an online cross-sectional survey designed to understand seafarers' behaviour and knowledge during COVID-19. A similar study was conducted on USA residents during the early epidemic phase to evaluate their knowledge levels and behavioural characteristics [18]. This study is among one of the first attempts to measure the knowledge on COVID-19 among crew members of merchant ships addressing requests for telemedical advice to the Centro Internazionale Radio Medico (C.I.R.M., International Radio Medical Centre).

2. Methods

2.1. Participants

The current cross-sectional investigation enlisted a sample of seafarers from the C.I.R.M. [19]. With more than 100,000 seafarers assisted onboard ships, the C.I.R.M. is the maritime telemedical centre with the largest experience of medical assistance to sailing seafarers. It was established in 1935 to give free radio medical advice to ships of all nationalities navigating in international waters. The C.I.R.M. is the Italian Telemedical Maritime Assistance Service (TMAS). The online questionnaire was delivered to 5000 seafarers, and 1458 (about 30%) agreed to provide consent to participate in this survey. We assumed that the participants that did not show interest in this study was due to a lack of internet onboard, staying with family because of fear caused by COVID-19, or a low-level knowledge of English.

2.2. Survey

The questionnaire included in the survey was refined by phrase changing, the possibility of adding new questions, and modifications of other research studies that provide extensive knowledge on the COVID-19 epidemic. Two C.I.R.M. doctors thoroughly reviewed the final questionnaire to make sure each item of the survey was clearly understood. The final questionnaire consisted of 25 questions and was distributed through a Google Form link.

The survey was organized into three sections: demographic characteristics, including age, rank onboard, members onboard, and educational status, etc. (5 items); personal characteristics (14 items); and the knowledge questionnaire had 6 questions regarding clinical presentation (2 questions), COVID-19 transmission routes (2 questions), and prevention and control (2 questions). Moreover, the questionnaire was adapted from previous studies on COVID-19 knowledge [18,20]. These questions were answered by correct and incorrect options. As a result, a correct answer was assigned "1", and an incorrect answer was assigned "0".

Before starting the survey, seafarers read an informed consent explanation that portrayed that cooperation was deliberate and that they could stop whenever. By tapping on a "next" button, members were considered as agreeing to finish the online questionnaire. The survey consisted of closed-ended questions, of which six permitted the seafarers to have the chance to give further details if the "other" alternative was chosen from the multiple-choice questions. The closed-ended questionnaire consisted of categorical, dichotomous, multiple-choice, and Likert-type questions on five-point rating scales. At the end of the questionnaire, we requested the participants provide final feedback regarding their participation in the study.

2.3. Reliability and Validity of Responses

The main objective of any questionnaire is to gather relevant information most reliably and validly. These factors are commonly associated with the conduction and selection of valid research instruments. As mentioned, this was a study related to onboard behavioural characteristics of seafarers, and we adopted the face validity method that was done by an analysis of the data using Cohen's Kappa Index (CKI). A kappa value that was greater than 0.6 was accepted as a valid question [21]. The items in the knowledge questionnaire were further validated with the CKI scale.

2.4. Statistical Analysis

Demographic variables such as age, rank, and educational status were done using frequency analysis. Frequencies of correct answers to knowledge questions were determined. A one-way analysis of variance (ANOVA) was used to determine the differences in the mean knowledge scores between the age groups, rank groups, and educational status. The t-test was used to understand the knowledge attitude differences to COVID-19 among different occupational groups of seafarers, and a p-value of ≤ 0.05 was considered statistically significant. Statistical analysis was carried out by IBM SPSS v.26 (Armonk, New York, NY, USA).

2.5. Ethical Approval

The review board members and the Ethics Committee of C.I.R.M. approved this study. The checklist for research ethics during the COVID pandemic was adopted from the UK research integrity office (UKRIO) guidelines [22]. This study was reviewed and approved by the C.I.R.M. Research Ethics Committee (ESI/2020/017). All participants provided consent by responding to a yes/no inquiry toward the beginning of the survey before they responded to the first question.

3. Results

Table 1 includes the participants' basic demographic characteristics: age group, rank onboard, and educational status. Table 2 presents nine questionnaires that were administered to measure the awareness about COVID-19, including clinical characteristics, transmission, prevention, and control. Among the total number of the respondents, the majority (97.87%) of them reported that they are aware of the novel coronavirus outbreak. Of the respondents that reported, 93.63% said that they were never infected by the new coronavirus, and 88.73% of the respondents reported that none of the people in their immediate social environments were infected.

Table 1. Participant demographic and awareness characteristics.

Demographic Characteristics	N	%
Gender		
Male	1241	85.11
Female	217	14.89
Age (Years)		
<20	21	1.4
20–30	332	22.8
30–40	431	29.6
40–50	571	39.2
>60	103	7.1
Education		
Primary education	44	1.01
College/University education	1237	92.82
Secondary School education	177	6.17
Rank on board		
Deck Officers	579	39.72
Deck Rating	281	19.24
Engine Officers	268	18.35
Engine Rating	220	15.11
Galley	111	7.58

Regarding behaviours, 42.57% of the participants reported that they were moving with other staff onboard, and just 0.22% of participants used a bed previously used by someone who got infected. Most seafarers (98.4%) provided a correct response on the transmission of the novel coronavirus. Regarding mental health status, 33 (2.24%) seafarers reported feeling lonely, 862 (59.13%) seafarers reported feeling well, 395 (27.10%) seafarers reported missing family/friends and 168 (11.53%) seafarers reported feeling overstressed.

The correct answers to knowledge questions ranged from 91.8% to 99.4% (Table 3). The mean COVID-19 knowledge score was 5.82 (standard deviation = 0.51, range 0–6), and the overall correct percentage was 97%. Most of the seafarers (99.4%) were aware of the COVID-19 clinical symptoms, and 95.7% realized that all infected individuals did not develop into severe cases. Viral infections are highly contagious among the people who live nearby and spread by respiratory droplets. Most respondents (97.3%) were aware that COVID-19 can be caused by human transmission when infected persons cough or sneeze.

Table 2. Awareness on COVID-19 onboard.

Q1. Are you aware of the novel coronavirus outbreak?		
Heard from Others	13	0.90
No	18	1.23
Yes	1427	97.87
Q2. Are you or have you been infected with the novel coronavirus?		
Do not know	86	5.92
No	1365	93.63
Yes, confirmed	7	0.45
Q3. Do you know people in your immediate social environment who are or have been infected with the novel coronavirus?		
Do not know	106	7.25
No	1294	88.73
Yes, confirmed	42	2.91
Yes, not confirmed	16	1.11
Q4. Are you closely moving with other staff onboard?		
No	196	13.41
Sometimes, I cannot avoid	642	44.02
Yes	621	42.57
Q5. Was your travel history associated with infected countries in the last two months?		
Maybe	52	3.58
No	414	28.41
Yes	992	68.01
Q6. Have you used a bed previously used by someone who got infected by coronavirus?		
May be	18	1.23
No	1436	98.5
Yes	3	0.22
Q7. Which of the following is correct about the transmission of the novel coronavirus?		
Do not know	11	0.78
The novel coronavirus is not transmissible	3	0.22
The novel coronavirus is transmissible from person to person.	1435	98.44
The novel coronavirus is transmitted by animals to humans only	8	0.56
Q8. Are your handwashing for at least 20 s?		
Yes	1366	93.68
No	92	6.32
Q9. How is your mental health during these periods		
Missing family and friends	395	27.1
Feeling lonely	33	2.24
More often getting stress	168	11.53
Feeling well	862	59.13

Table 3. Frequency of correct answers to the knowledge questions. CKI: Cohen's Kappa Index.

Knowledge Questions	N (Correct%)	CKI
KQ1: The main clinical symptoms of COVID-19 are fever, fatigue, shortness of breath, and dry cough.	1449 (99.4)	0.7
KQ2: Not all persons with COVID-19 will develop into severe cases. Those who are older and have chronic illnesses such as diabetes, heart diseases, cancer, and chronic kidney diseases are more likely to have severe cases.	1395 (95.7)	0.6
KQ3: The COVID-19 virus spreads via respiratory droplets of infected individuals.	1418 (97.3)	0.8
KQ4: By wearing masks onboard, it is possible to control the speed of the virus spreading.	1338 (91.8)	0.9
KQ5: Isolations and treatment of people who are infected with COVID-19 are effective ways to reduce the spread of the virus.	1443 (99)	0.8
KQ6: People who have contact with someone infected with the COVID-19 virus should be immediately isolated. In general, the observation period is 14 days.	1448 (99.3)	0.7

Based on the guidelines provided by the World Health Organization (WHO), it is evident that wearing facemasks only can help prevent becoming infected with the virus [23]. In this study, 92% of participants agreed that spreading of the virus can be controlled by wearing masks onboard; 99% mentioned that treatment and isolation are promising ways to reduce the virus transmission, and 99.3% provided the correct response on the incubation period of COVID-19. These findings appreciate the well-known knowledge of emphasizing maintaining onboard social distancing to control further infections. There was a statistically significant difference between the age groups ($F_{(4, 1453)} = 5.44$, $p < 0.001$) and rank groups ($F_{(4, 1453)} = 32.18$, $p < 0.001$), as determined by one-way ANOVA. The knowledge scores were not significantly different across the educational statuses of the participants ($F_{(2, 1455)} = 1.52$, $p = 0.220$) (Table 4).

Table 4. Background characteristics of seafarers and knowledge scores of COVID-19 by age, rank, and educational status.

	Demographic Characteristics			
	N (%)	Knowledge (Mean + S.D)	F-Test	p-Value
Age Group				
<20 Years	21 (1.44)	5.43 + 0.81		
20–30 Years	312 (21.4)	5.76 + 0.56		
31–40 Years	440 (30.2)	5.84 + 0.49	5.44	<0.001
41–50 Years	573 (39.3)	5.86 + 0.44		
>51 Years	112 (7.7)	5.79 + 0.60		
Rank category				
Deck officer	579 (39.7)	5.98 + 0.12		
Engine officer	268 (18.4)	5.76 + 0.57		
Deck Rating	281 (19.3)	5.73 + 0.61	32.18	0.220
Engine Rating	220 (15)	5.74 + 0.60		
Galley	110 (7.5)	5.51 + 0.76		
Educational status				
Primary school	44 (3)	5.70 + 0.55		
Secondary school	177 (12)	5.85 + 0.45	1.52	<0.001
College/University	1237 (85)	5.82 + 0.52		

The data on the knowledge of daily preventive measures by seafarers are summarized in Figure 1. As shown, few respondents had limited knowledge due to a low educational status. Among the total respondents, 1412 (97%) indicated that they avoid face touching,

1347 (92.38%) anticipated covering their faces when they sneezed or coughed, and 986 (68%) chose disinfectants for cleaning their hands when soap was not available. Moreover, 1226 (84%) followed social distancing onboard, and 1128 (77.3%) wore masks while moving onboard. To increase their immune systems, 801 (55%) preferred to do exercise, 481 (33%) habitually drank ginger tea, and only 47 (3%) were interested in using antibiotics.

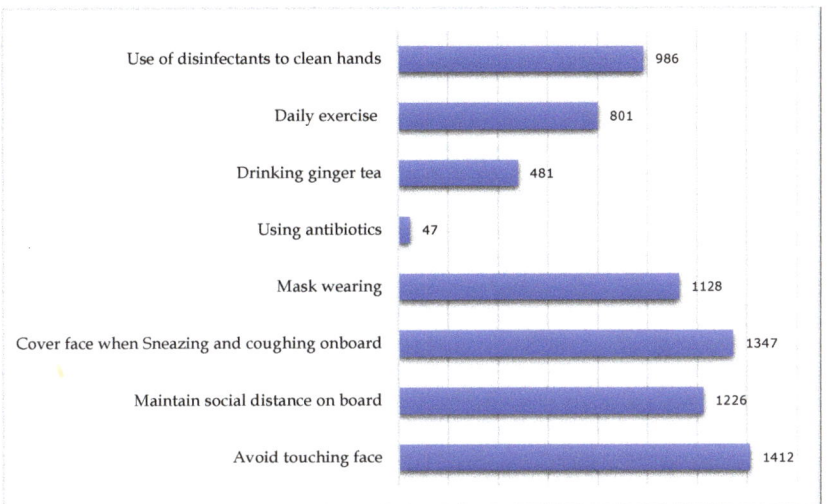

Figure 1. Onboard individual prevention measures by seafarers.

4. Discussion

Many studies were found related to the knowledge, attitudes, and practices (KAP) concerning the COVID-19 outbreak [24–27], but the literature search did not identify any works on seafarer COVID-19 knowledge assessments. Due to this, we developed a tool to investigate COVID-19 knowledge, including behavioural characteristics and the necessity of onboard health measures.

4.1. Personal Awareness

The personal awareness questionnaire was created to understand the factors that decide virus transmission onboard and further classified into three constructs, such as environment hygiene, socio-travel characteristics, and poor health literacy. These, indeed, are considered the four factors that demonstrate seafarers' knowledge of COVID-19 transmission.

Early data on public health practices embraced to forestall the spread of COVID-19 might help control the virus transmission; it is also necessary to publicize knowledge of the psychological characteristics of the stigma and social discrimination (SAD) in pandemic realities [28,29]. Recent evidence confirmed that the COVID-19 disease is transmitted by either physical contact or respiratory droplets of an infected person [30]. Moreover, contact transmission can be possible when an infected individual onboard touch their nose, eye, or mouth mucosa, and the virus can also be transferred from one surface to another by contaminated hands. Due to this, hand hygiene is mandatory to prevent the COVID-19 virus spread. In this study, 97.3% of seafarers agreed with the concept that the virus spread was caused by respiratory droplets of contaminated individuals. Rubbing hands with alcohol-based soap for at least 20 s is an effective approach to neutralize viruses like corona because of an oily surface membrane that is decomposed by soap [31]. The highest number (93.68%) of seafarers mentioned that they do 20-s hand washes with alcoholic soaps.

Travel behaviour is another important characteristic of the spread of COVID in any working culture. Due to global trading during the pandemic, the percentage of the population engaged in international travel is higher in Western countries like Europe, the USA, and others. In the present study, 992 (68.01%) seafarers mentioned that they travelled to infected nations during April and May 2020. Moreover, COVID-19 can largely spread among the populations of infected cases in the next social environment [32]. Respondents mentioned that about 58 (4%) people were suspected of contracting COVID-19 during working conditions, and 42 members were confirmed as infected. Maintaining social distancing with other employees also prevents the virus spread, but sometimes, it is hard to avoid staff movements in closed environments. 40% of participants mentioned that they are aware of social distancing but are unable to escape from unexpected situations, and 42.57% are closely moving with others. Maintain isolation onboard for people who are confirmed or suspected by COVID-19. A person in isolation is not supposed to leave the place and keep away from the public on the ship. Others should also be aware of not sharing the belongings of infected people. Most of the seafarers (98.5%) did not intend to use the bed of a COVID-19-infected person.

Poor health literacy about COVID-19 is an underrated global public health issue. Significant health literacy already seems like an important tool for the prevention of non-communicable diseases like an ongoing epidemic [33]. In the present research, 97.87% of members said that they were aware of the present virus outbreak, and 98.44% of respondents were well informed about it being caused by human transmission.

4.2. Seafarers' COVID-19 Knowledge

COVID-19 is an ongoing pandemic with serious threats to public health [34]. Since most of the vaccines are under trails, preventive measures are the only solution to control it, and therefore, everyone should have minimum knowledge on this novel virus. Attempts to change behaviours are basic in limiting the easy transmission of diseases like COVID-19, and it is unclear whether people knew about the risk of disease and adjusted their behaviours during the early times of the pandemic [35]. Due to its highly contagious nature in enclosed areas, seafarers' behaviours on a ship are probably the main factor in deciding the spread of a COVID-19 epidemic. Their behaviours are affected by their perceptions and individual knowledge.

The study outcomes indicated that most of the seafarers were knowledgeable, and respondents achieved a mean of 97% in the knowledge questionnaire. This value is higher than other audiences, like the general public and health workers, which ranged from 62% to 81.4% [24–27]. In this study, the 92.82% rate of correct answers is probably related to the cultural background of the respondents that mostly had a college or university education. This is also due to the time that the questionnaire distribution happened during the virus outbreak. During this time, seafarers already gained some knowledge regarding COVID-19 prevention and transmission causes via the internet, media platforms, or colleague discussions. The close associations found among educational background, age, and knowledge ($p < 0.001$) supports our claims. On the other hand, the knowledge of daily preventive measures by seafarers was much appreciable. Very few respondents had limited knowledge due to a low educational status.

In terms of the seafarers' behavioural characteristics on ships, the respondents presented a positive and encouraging approach towards COVID-19. About 96% agreed that the virus does not develop into a serious illness unless in the presence of other chronic diseases. These inspirational mentalities and high trust in the control of COVID-19 can be clarified by the marine industries' phenomenal activities and brief reaction times for taking tough control and prudent steps against COVID-19 to defend ship workers and guarantee their better health. These measures include isolation, avoid travelling on other ships, regulations on mask-wearing, and sanitization of the workplace regularly.

4.3. Study Strengths and Limitations

This is probably the first study that investigated the awareness and knowledge regarding COVID-19 among the seafarer population. The data collection involved nearly

30 shipping companies, including more than 1,000 ship workers. The preliminary results encourage ship authorities to provide explicit guidelines and plan preventive actions to avoid the future spread of the virus at ship working places. Despite the promising knowledge outcomes, the present study had some limitations. Since the data analysis was conducted with the help of a self-reported questionnaire, there is a chance of biased outcomes. Forthcoming works must use administrative questionnaire data to overcome this issue. Besides, community-based sample (like seafarers) studies cannot provide as much evidence on the severity of pandemics as the data collected through participants of author networks. On the other hand, the highest number of participants were from European shipping companies, and future research needs to include worldwide merchant ship members.

5. Conclusions

The current global pandemic caused by the COVID-19 disease is creating awful situations for both seafarers and marine industries. By maintaining a close relationship between shipping companies, flag and port states, and others, maritime service providers can protect seafarers' health and, simultaneously, the public [36]. Certain web-based interventions like online questionnaires can enhance the individual knowledge of seafarers by informing, educating, reminding, and monitoring to fight against the ongoing epidemic. Hygiene conditions, waste management, and room sanitation onboard are mandatory to protect an individual's health during virus outbreaks, including COVID-19. Guaranteeing continuous handwashing and practices in waste management at working stations will help to control the person-to-person transmission of the virus. This study was conducted during the COVID-19 first wave, and we would like to recontact the participants to evaluate their behaviours at the surge of the present second wave. Alternatively, telemedicine represents the most realistic approach to provide medical assistance at sea. The same technologies respecting legal and ethical standards [37] should be considered for providing health education of seafarers.

Author Contributions: Conceptualization, G.B. and G.G.S.; methodology, G.B.; software, G.B.; validation, G.B., G.G.S. and M.D.C.; formal analysis, G.B.; investigation, G.B.; resources, G.B.; data curation, G.B., N.C. and G.G.S.; writing—original draft preparation, G.B. and F.A.; writing—review and editing, G.B.; visualization, G.B. and M.D.C.; supervision, F.A.; project administration, F.A.; funding acquisition, F.A. All authors have read and agreed to the published version of the manuscript.

Funding: This study was supported by the ITF Trust grant No. 1508/2020 to the Centro Internationale Radio Medico (C.I.R.M.). Institutional funding of the University of Camerino, Italy, supported this work. G.B., G.G.S., and N.C. were recipients of PhD bursaries from the University of Camerino.

Institutional Review Board Statement: The study was conducted according to the guidelines of the Declaration of UK research integrity office (UKRIO) during COVID-19 by the Ethics Committee of C.I.R.M.

Informed Consent Statement: Informed consent was obtained from all subjects involved in the study.

Data Availability Statement: The COVID-19 data were extracted from the public domain data repository of the Centre for Systems Science and Engineering (CSSE) at John Hopkins University.

Acknowledgments: The collaboration of the Italian Shipowners associations Confitarma and Assarmatori in promoting participation in the survey is gratefully acknowledged. The authors are indebted to A Saturnino (C.I.R.M., Rome) for his support in the distribution of the questionnaire.

Conflicts of Interest: No author does not have any conflict of interest.

References

1. Huang, C.; Wang, Y.; Li, X.; Ren, L.; Zhao, J.; Hu, Y.; Zhang, L.; Fan, G.; Xu, J.; Gu, X.; et al. Clinical features of patients infected with 2019 novel coronavirus in Wuhan, China. *Lancet* **2020**, *395*, 497–506. [CrossRef]
2. COVID-19 Map—Johns Hopkins Coronavirus Resource Center. Available online: https://coronavirus.jhu.edu/map.html (accessed on 5 January 2021).

3. Battineni, G.; Chintalapudi, N.; Amenta, F. AI Chatbot Design during an Epidemic like the Novel Coronavirus. *Healthcare* **2020**, *8*, 154. [CrossRef]
4. Bontempi, E. The europe second wave of COVID-19 infection and the Italy "strange" situation. *Environ. Res.* **2020**, 110476. [CrossRef] [PubMed]
5. Chintalapudi, N.; Battineni, G.; Amenta, F. COVID-19 virus outbreak forecasting of registered and recovered cases after sixty day lockdown in Italy: A data driven model approach. *J. Microbiol. Immunol. Infect.* **2020**, *53*, 396–403. [CrossRef] [PubMed]
6. Sawano, T.; Ozaki, A.; Rodriguez-Morales, A.J.; Tanimoto, T.; Sah, R. Limiting spread of COVID-19 from cruise ships: Lessons to be learnt from Japan. *QJM Int. J. Med.* **2020**, *113*, 309–310. [CrossRef] [PubMed]
7. Mizumoto, K.; Kagaya, K.; Zarebski, A.; Chowell, G. Estimating the asymptomatic proportion of coronavirus disease 2019 (COVID-19) cases on board the Diamond Princess cruise ship, Yokohama, Japan, 2020. *Eurosurveillance* **2020**, *25*, 2000180. [CrossRef]
8. Malone, J.D. USS Theodore Roosevelt, COVID-19, and Ships: Lessons Learned. *JAMA Netw. Open* **2020**, *3*, e2022095. [CrossRef]
9. Fernandes, E.G.; Santos, J.D.S.; Sato, H.K. Outbreak investigation in cargo ship in times of COVID-19 crisis, Port of Santos, Brazil. *Rev. Saúde Pública* **2020**, *54*, 34. [CrossRef]
10. International Labour Standards on Seafarers. Available online: https://www.ilo.org/global/standards/subjects-covered-by-international-labour-standards/seafarers/lang--en/index.htm (accessed on 8 January 2021).
11. International Maritime Orgnization Home Page. Available online: https://www.imo.org/en (accessed on 6 January 2021).
12. Battineni, G.; Amenta, F. Designing of an Expert system for the management of Seafarer's health. *Digit. Health* **2020**, *6*. [CrossRef]
13. Sagaro, G.G.; Battineni, G.; Chintalapudi, N.; Di Canio, M.; Amenta, F. Telemedicine assistance at sea in the time of COVID-19 pandemic. *Int. Marit. Health* **2020**, *71*, 229–236. [CrossRef]
14. COVID-19 Vaccines. Available online: https://www.who.int/emergencies/diseases/novel-coronavirus-2019/covid-19-vaccines (accessed on 5 January 2021).
15. Coronavirus Hits More Cruise Ships, Leaving Vessels Stuck at Sea—WSJ. Available online: https://www.wsj.com/articles/coronavirus-hits-more-cruise-ships-leaving-vessels-stuck-at-sea-11584373335 (accessed on 5 January 2021).
16. Battineni, G.; Chintalapudi, N.; Amenta, F. SARS-CoV-2 epidemic calculation in Italy by SEIR compartmental models. *Appl. Comput. Inform.* **2020**. [CrossRef]
17. Haghani, M.; Bliemer, M.C.; Goerlandt, F.; Li, J. The scientific literature on Coronaviruses, COVID-19 and its associated safety-related research dimensions: A scientometric analysis and scoping review. *Saf. Sci.* **2020**, *129*, 104806. [CrossRef] [PubMed]
18. Clements, J.M. Knowledge and Behaviors toward COVID-19 among US Residents during the Early Days of the Pandemic: Cross-Sectional Online Questionnaire. *J. Med. Internet Res.* **2020**, *6*, e19161. [CrossRef] [PubMed]
19. Battineni, G.; Sagaro, G.G.; Chintalapudi, N.; Amenta, F. Conceptual Framework and Designing for a Seafarers' Health Observatory (SHO) Based on the Centro Internazionale Radio Medico (C.I.R.M.) Data Repository. *Sci. World J.* **2020**, *2020*, 1–5. [CrossRef] [PubMed]
20. Ferdous, M.Z.; Islam, S.; Sikder, T.; Mosaddek, A.S.M.; Zegarra-Valdivia, J.A.; Gozal, D. Knowledge, attitude, and practice regarding COVID-19 outbreak in Bangladesh: An online-based cross-sectional study. *PLoS ONE* **2020**, *15*, e0239254. [CrossRef] [PubMed]
21. Taherdoost, H. Validity and Reliability of the Research Instrument; How to Test the Validation of a Questionnaire/Survey in a Research. *SSRN Electron. J.* **2018**. [CrossRef]
22. UKRIO. Checklist during COVID-19. Available online: https://ukrio.org/publications/recommended-checklist-during-covid-19/ (accessed on 10 January 2021).
23. WHO. Mask Use in the Context of COVID-19, Who, No. December 2020, pp. 1–10. Available online: https://www.who.int/publications/i/item/advice-on-the-use-of-masks-in-the-community-during-home-care-and-in-healthcare-settings-in-the-context-of-the-novel-coronavirus-(2019-ncov)-outbreak (accessed on 1 January 2021).
24. Zhong, B.L.; Luo, W.; Li, H.M.; Zhang, Q.Q.; Liu, X.G.; Li, W.T.; Li, Y. Knowledge, attitudes, and practices towards COVID-19 among Chinese residents during the rapid rise period of the COVID-19 outbreak: A quick online cross-sectional survey. *Int. J. Biol. Sci.* **2020**, *16*, 1745–1752. [CrossRef]
25. Al-Hanawi, M.K.; Angawi, K.; Alshareef, N.; Qattan, A.M.N.; Helmy, H.Z.; Abudawood, Y.; AlQurashi, M.; Kattan, W.M.; Kadasah, N.A.; Chirwa, G.C.; et al. Knowledge, Attitude and Practice Toward COVID-19 Among the Public in the Kingdom of Saudi Arabia: A Cross-Sectional Study. *Front. Public Health* **2020**, *8*, 217. [CrossRef]
26. Azlan, A.A.; Hamzah, M.R.; Sern, T.J.; Ayub, S.H.; Mohamad, E.M. Public knowledge, attitudes and practices towards COVID-19: A cross-sectional study in Malaysia. *PLoS ONE* **2020**, *15*, e0233668. [CrossRef]
27. Akalu, Y.; Ayelign, B.; Molla, M.D. Knowledge, Attitude and Practice towards COVID-19 among Chronic Disease Patients at Addis Zemen Hospital, Northwest Ethiopia. *Infect. Drug Resist.* **2020**, *13*, 1949–1960. [CrossRef]
28. Irigoyen-Camacho, M.E.; Velazquez-Alva, M.C.; Zepeda-Zepeda, M.A.; Cabrer-Rosales, M.F.; Lazarevich, I.; Castaño-Seiquer, A. Effect of Income Level and Perception of Susceptibility and Severity of COVID-19 on Stay-at-Home Preventive Behavior in a Group of Older Adults in Mexico City. *Int. J. Environ. Res. Public Health* **2020**, *17*, 7418. [CrossRef] [PubMed]
29. Baldassarre, A.; Giorgi, G.; Alessio, F.; Lulli, L.G.; Arcangeli, G.; Mucci, N. Stigma and Discrimination (SAD) at the Time of the SARS-CoV-2 Pandemic. *Int. J. Environ. Res. Public Health* **2020**, *17*, 6341. [CrossRef] [PubMed]

30. Dhand, R.; Li, J. Coughs and Sneezes: Their Role in Transmission of Respiratory Viral Infections, Including SARS-CoV-2. *Am. J. Respir. Crit. Care Med.* **2020**, *202*, 651–659. [CrossRef] [PubMed]
31. WHO. *Updated WHO Recommendations for International Traffic in Relation to COVID-19 Outbreak, COVID-19 Travel Advice*; WHO: Geneva, Switzerland, 2020.
32. Chintalapudi, N.; Battineni, G.; Sagaro, G.G.; Amenta, F. COVID-19 outbreak reproduction number estimations and forecasting in Marche, Italy. *Int. J. Infect. Dis.* **2020**, *96*, 327–333. [CrossRef]
33. Nguyen, H.C.; Nguyen, M.H.; Do, B.N.; Tran, C.Q.; Nguyen, T.T.P.; Pham, K.M.; Pham, L.V.; Tran, K.V.; Duong, T.T.; Tran, T.V.; et al. People with Suspected COVID-19 Symptoms Were More Likely Depressed and Had Lower Health-Related Quality of Life: The Potential Benefit of Health Literacy. *J. Clin. Med.* **2020**, *9*, 965. [CrossRef]
34. Dryhurst, S.; Schneider, C.R.; Kerr, J.R.; Freeman, A.L.J.; Recchia, G.; Van Der Bles, A.M.; Spiegelhalter, D.; Van Der Linden, S. Risk perceptions of COVID-19 around the world. *J. Risk Res.* **2020**, *23*, 994–1006. [CrossRef]
35. Wise, T.; Zbozinek, T.D.; Michelini, G.; Hagan, C.C.; Mobbs, D. Changes in risk perception and self-reported protective behaviour during the first week of the COVID-19 pandemic in the United States: COVID-19 risk perception and behavior. *R. Soc. Open Sci.* **2020**. [CrossRef]
36. Ipsema | Facile.it. Available online: https://www.facile.it/assicurazioni/glossario/ipsema.html (accessed on 10 January 2021).
37. Nittari, G.; Khuman, R.; Baldoni, S.; Pallotta, G.; Battineni, G.; Sirignano, A.; Amenta, F.; Ricci, G. Telemedicine Practice: Review of the Current Ethical and Legal Challenges. *Telemed. J. E-Health* **2020**, *26*, 1427–1437. [CrossRef]

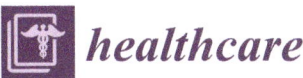

Article

Prevention and Control of COVID-19 Pandemic on International Cruise Ships: The Legal Controversies

Xiaohan Zhang [1] and Chao Wang [2,*]

[1] Guanghua Law School, Zhejiang University, Hangzhou 310008, China; zhangxiaohan@zju.edu.cn
[2] Academy of International Strategy and Law, Zhejiang University, Hangzhou 310008, China
* Correspondence: zjuwang@yeah.net

Abstract: During the COVID-19 pandemic in 2020, a number of international cruise ships were infected, thereby resulting in serious public health and human rights problems. Multiple difficulties were encountered in the prevention and control of the coronavirus disease onboard ships, while rule-based international cooperation in this regard appeared inefficient and ineffective. By applying interdisciplinary methodologies, including empirical research of law, policy science, and health studies, this research reviewed the legal difficulties in the prevention and control of COVID-19 on international cruise ships and sought solutions from a policy-making and strategic perspective. We found that, apart from the inherent nature of cruise ships such as crowded semi-enclosed areas, shared sanitary facilities and limited medical resources, there are also nonnegligible legal reasons affecting the effectiveness of containment measures on board. In particular, there is ambiguity and even inconsistency of relevant international norms and domestic regulations, and some of the key rules are neither mandatory nor enforceable. We conclude by suggesting that rule-based international cooperation on this issue must be strengthened with respect to information sharing and management, a more effective supervisory mechanism, clarification of key rules over jurisdiction and distributions of obligations among the port states, flag states, nationality states, and cruise ship companies.

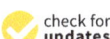

Citation: Zhang, X.; Wang, C. Prevention and Control of COVID-19 Pandemic on International Cruise Ships: The Legal Controversies. *Healthcare* **2021**, *9*, 281. https://doi.org/10.3390/healthcare9030281

Academic Editors: Manoj Sharma and Kavita Batra

Received: 2 February 2021
Accepted: 1 March 2021
Published: 4 March 2021

Publisher's Note: MDPI stays neutral with regard to jurisdictional claims in published maps and institutional affiliations.

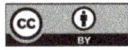

Copyright: © 2021 by the authors. Licensee MDPI, Basel, Switzerland. This article is an open access article distributed under the terms and conditions of the Creative Commons Attribution (CC BY) license (https://creativecommons.org/licenses/by/4.0/).

Keywords: COVID-19; infectious disease; international cruises; health policy and regulation; control strategies; international cooperation; global health governance

1. Introduction

International cruise tourism is the fastest growing sector of the travel industry since the early 1990s. Statistics show that in the past decade, cruising around the world has continued to boom with an average annual growth rate of 6.8 percent, and it was estimated that in 2020 the global ocean cruise industry would carry over 32 million passengers [1]. However, the sudden outbreak of COVID-19 at the end of 2019 deeply impacted this $150 billion industry as a number of international cruise ships were infected. The British-registered Diamond Princess cruise ship was the first one to have a major onboard outbreak, with over 700 people being infected, and the ship being quarantined at the Yokohama port of Japan on 4 February 2020, for nearly one month. By the end of May 2020, over 40 cruise ships had confirmed coronavirus cases. The last infected cruise ship with passengers onboard during the first wave of COVID-19, the German-based Artania, docked at its home port with its last passengers on 8 June 2020 [2]. During this period, many countries closed their borders and blocked international cruise ships from docking in order to prevent and control the pandemic. The United States Centers for Disease Control and Prevention (CDC), for instance, issued a No Sail Order effective on 13 March 2020 that suspended all cruise ship passenger operations [3]. As a consequence, thousands of passengers were quarantined on board for weeks before coming ashore, while seafarers were trapped at sea for an even longer time before being repatriated, resulting in "a humanitarian, safety and economic crisis" as described by the International Maritime Organization (IMO) [4].

Outbreaks of COVID-19 on international cruise ships attracted worldwide concern not only from stakeholders including cruise lines and national governments but also from researchers and the public. As a matter of fact, due to the inherent features of cruise ships such as the high population density, shared food supplies, and semi-enclosed living environments, the spread of infectious diseases occurs relatively easily on board [5]. There is scientific evidence in existing epidemiological studies suggesting that respiratory diseases, including influenza, legionnaires' disease, avian influenza A(H7N9) and Middle East Respiratory Syndrome (MERS), are all among the most dangerous and high-risk viruses on cruise ships [6,7]. Once such infectious diseases break out on board, the viruses usually transmit rapidly and lead to public health emergencies that pose substantial challenges to the safety of ports and coastal states. During the COVID-19 pandemic, there is clear evidence that passengers aboard cruise ships played a role in spreading the coronavirus disease to a number of countries [8].

Both the prevention and the control of infectious diseases on cruise ships are relatively more complicated and problematic, especially for those international ships with passengers of different nationalities and docking ports located in different countries. Apart from the limited healthcare and medical conditions onboard, there are also difficulties with respect to the rule-based international cooperation and coordination of treatment measures. During the first wave of the COVID-19 pandemic, a number of international cruise ships were denied from docking or entering into the costal ports, as states applied different, changing, and sometimes even conflicting rules. The Holland America *MS Westerdam* cruise ship is a typical case in point. After departing from Hong Kong with 1455 passengers and 802 crew members on 1 February 2020, because of suspected coronavirus cases on board, the ship was denied entry not only by its destination port of Yokohama but also by other nearby ports in Japan, South Korea, Guam, Thailand, and the Philippines. On 13 February 2020, the ship was finally accepted by Sihanoukville Port in Cambodia, ending its two weeks' helplessly drifting at sea. From a legal perspective, do these states have the right to deny entry? Which state is obligated to provide assistance in a public health emergency? If an infected ship is permitted to dock and disembark passengers, what measures can the port state take under its governing laws? How can it be ensured that all involved parties, including the flag state, the coastal state, and the ship operator/owner's state, will cooperate effectively in the face of a global pandemic? All these issues are important for international cruise ships to prevent and control the on-going COVID-19 pandemic. However, they largely remain unclear and even unanswered. Existing literature and research mainly focus on textual interpretation of relevant legal provisions under normal circumstances, but without concurrently taking into account the unique features of international cruise ships. Much less is discussed under the on-going COVID-19 pandemic circumstance, which have brought upon unprecedented new challenges to the whole world.

Against this backdrop, this research article aims to analyze the international regulatory issues relating to the prevention and control of epidemics on international cruise ships, with a special focus on investigating those legal mechanisms from the perspective of strategies and policies of epidemic prevention and control. Section 2 introduces the collection of data, research materials, and methods of this research. Section 3 presents the research findings about the various legal difficulties of preventing and controlling COVID-19 on international cruise ships, and briefly summarizes the legal issues and conclusions. Section 4 further analyzes and discusses those regulatory issues in detail. Section 5 provides suggestions for addressing the aforementioned issues.

2. Materials and Methods

2.1. Research Data

Regarding the facts about outbreaks of the COVID-19 pandemic on international cruise ships, relevant information and data were collected mainly through the official websites of involved institutions, such as the International Maritime Organization (IMO), the

International Cruise Line Association (ICLA), and other public sources such as Wikipedia and international news reports. The searching period for the factual data is set between January 2020 and December 2020.

For policies and strategies of COVID-19 prevention and control on cruise ships, research materials and data were collected mainly through relevant governmental departments, such as Japan's Ministry of Health, Labour and Welfare, China's National Health Committee and Maritime Safety Administration, and the United States Centers for Disease Control and Prevention (CDC) as well as its Vessel Sanitation Program (VSP). For academic analysis and discussions of these policies and strategies, research literature and references were obtained by searching databases such as PubMed, Medline, and Embase using keywords cruise ships, infectious disease, COVID-19, travel health, ship sanitation, and PHEIC.

For research questions on the governing laws and precedent cases, such as the interpretation and application of relevant provisions of the United Nations Convention on the Law of the Sea (UNCLOS), the WHO's International Health Regulations (IHR), and the IMO's Guidelines on Places of Refuge for Ships in Need of Assistance, references were acquired by searching Heinonline, Westlaw, LexisNexis and other professional legal databases.

2.2. Research Methods

Interdisciplinary methodologies including empirical research of law, policy science, and health studies were adopted. The comprehensive search and literature review of COVID-19 cases that are linked to cruise ships were conducted so as to provide a strong basis for empirical analysis and further discussions. Past public health incidents on international cruise ships during other pandemics such as SARS and MERS are also referred to. Based on findings of these facts, the actual effects of relevant rule-based mechanisms on tackling cruise ships' public health emergencies are evaluated. These empirical studies will facilitate our understanding on the functioning of relevant legal regime and its impact on the formulation of pandemic control policies in the face of the COVID-19.

Doctrinal research, named "black letter" methodology, is fundamental to the study of legal issues. We will identify, describe, and critically analyze the text of relevant legal provisions contained in the UNCLOS, the IHR, and other relevant international conventions, as well as relevant domestic regulations of Japan, the United States, and other countries. The aim of textual analysis is to explore the original intention of legislation and identify ambiguities, inefficiencies, and even inconsistencies in relevant rules, based on which improvement suggestions and solutions are provided.

Case studies are also important for this research. We particularly focused on those representative cases such as the Diamond Princess cruise ship, which is considered a de facto epidemiological laboratory during the first wave of COVID-19 outbreaks in 2020. Lessons learned from this high-profile case are worth carefully studying in terms of strengthening rule-based international cooperation and improving health conditions on future cruise ships in similar pandemic situations. Major questions of these case studies include emerging regulatory issues encountered by various parties, whether and to what extent they are liable, whether their measures comply with relevant international and national norms and whether the right to health of people on board is sufficiently protected.

3. Results

Through data retrieval and analysis, we found that there was a COVID-19 pandemic outbreak on nearly 50 international cruise ships. A number of typical cases are listed in Table 1 below, which clearly indicates the complexity of this issue [9]. We also found that different cruise ships, ports, and coastal states adopted different measures to prevent and control the pandemic, which directly led to controversies. In particular, many ports were closed for travel restrictions and denied entry to international cruise ships and foreign nationals. Some countries such as Australia and the United States banned all foreign flagged ships from docking and directed them to leave, making no allowance for disembarkation.

As a consequence of these controversial measures, thousands of passengers and crew members around the world were stranded on board and unable to be repatriated home.

Table 1. List of selected COVID-19 cases on cruise ships.

Ship Name	Passenger	Crew	Cases	Dock/Location	Owner/Operator
Artania	800	500	89	Fremantle, Australia	Phoenix Reisen, German
Braemar	682	38	5	Mariel, Cuba	FOCL, Norway
Coral Princess	1020	878	12	Miami, USA	Princess Cruises, Bermuda
Costa Luminosa	1370	410	36	Marseille-Fos, France	Costa Cruises, Italy
Costa Magica	2309	945	2	Miami, USA	Costa Cruises, Italy
Diamond Princess	2666	1045	712	Yokohama, Japan	Princess Cruises, Bermuda
Grand Princess	2422	1111	122	Oakland, USA	Princess Cruises, Bermuda
Paul Gauguin	148	192	1	Papeete, France	Ponant, France
River Anuket	101	70	45	Luxor, Egypt	Holland America, USA
Roald Amundsen	177	160	36	Tromsø, Norway	Hurtigruten, Norway
Silver Shadow	318	291	2	Recife, Brazil	Royal Caribbean, USA
Westerdam	781	747	1	Sihanoukville, Cambodia	Holland America, USA
World Dream	1871	1820	12	Hong Kong, China	Dream Cruises, China
Zaandam	1243	586	11	Everglades, USA	Holland America, USA

The factors resulting in the difficulties of COVID-19 prevention and control on international cruise ships, apart from those inherent physical circumstances such as close living and working conditions and medical treatment restrictions on board, we found that the inadequacy and even failure of cooperation by involved parties were incredibly salient. The WHO has indicated that health on international cruise ships is a shared responsibility of all relevant stakeholders, involving equitable access to essential care and collective defense against transnational threats [10]. In terms of international cooperation when there is a Public Health Emergency of International Concern (PHEIC), ideally, all involved parties and states could make effort to cooperate with each other, whether for humanitarian purposes or to fulfill a specific obligation. During the first wave of the COVID-19 pandemic, we found that the fundamental international cooperation was weak. By taking cooperation under the United Nations framework as an example, although there are several specialized agencies such as the WHO, the ILO, and the IMO that are closely connected with the prevention and control of COVID-19 on international cruise ships, cooperation among them remains largely at the level of making joint declarations, with few joint actions. As a result, the functioning of these key international organizations appears inefficient and ineffective in the face of the COVID-19 pandemic.

We further found complicated legal motivations, as all measures and cooperation are rule-based. A large number and variety of laws and regulations, both national and international, are applicable to the issue of prevention and control of COVID-19 on international cruise ships. The UNCLOS, the foremost international agreement on law of the sea, for example, provides rules including the general obligation of maritime rescue and cooperation, jurisdiction of port states and flag states. Meanwhile, more substantial regulations on the management of ships and ports, entry and exit control, and health and quarantine requirements are contained and scattered in other international and national laws of the countries involved. In this regard, we discovered that there are certain ambiguity and even inconsistency with regard to the relevant international norms and the domestic regulations of individual states. Such a lack of regulatory harmony directly led to problems of conflicted jurisdictions, unbalanced liabilities, and an uncertainty of rescue obligations during the COVID-19 pandemic.

Moreover, some key rules are not enforceable or mandatory. For example, in order to cope with coastal states' prohibition of environmentally threatening foreign ships from entering their ports, the IMO passed two resolutions to address the issue of places of refuge for ships in distress: the Guidelines on Places of Refuge for Ships in Need of Assistance [11] and the Maritime Assistance Services [12], which contain provisions for the coastal states to establish a ship refuge system. Nevertheless, these norms are soft law in nature and are not mandatory for implementation by any party. Under the PHEIC circumstances, in consideration of other factors such as self-safety, high risks and costs, environment protection and even geopolitics, most coastal states are understandably disinclined to accept infected ships entering their refuge areas. As a consequence, those distressed ships usually could not be timely and efficiently rescued. Similarly, we found that another key international organization, the WHO, only has limited legislative and enforcement power to regulate epidemic control measures on international cruise ships, while most of its IHR provisions serve more as guidelines for the national governments. The free pratique principle and restrictions on it is a case in point in terms of implementing the IHR regulations during the COVID-19 pandemic.

4. Discussion

4.1. Free Pratique, Rescue Obligation, and Refusal of Entry

4.1.1. Application of the Free Pratique Principle

As a general principle, according to the IHR, a country shall grant ships the right of free pratique; that is, ships shall not be prevented from calling at any point of entry for public health reasons [13]. This is also in line with relevant UNCLOS provisions which require the coastal states to recognize the right of innocent passage for foreign ships [14]. Therefore, at the early stage of the COVID-19 outbreak, the WHO together with the IMO had called on all countries to respect the free pratique principle when noticing that several international cruise ships either experienced delayed port clearance or were denied entry to ports because of the coronavirus [15].

A limitation to the free pratique principle is that, when infection or contamination sources are found on board, a country may require disinfection, decontamination, disinsection or deratting, or other necessary measures that should be taken to prevent the spread of the infection or contamination [13]. The IHR also authorizes a country to take additional health measures pursuant to its national law, given that such measures are based on scientific principles, available scientific evidence of risk to human health, and the specific guidance or advice from the WHO [16]. Accordingly, a justified decision on whether there is a risk to human health requires actual and reliable research data; otherwise, the additional measures taken by an individual country will likely be challenged by other parties for lacking necessary evidence. This is the underlying reason why controversies arose when, during the COVID-19 pandemic, international cruise ships were denied entry into a number of costal states without justifications. For application of the "free pratique" principle, despite the insufficiencies of implementing relevant IHR provisions, whether a cruise ship might result in the spread of the coronavirus or bring other risks to the coastal states needs to be assessed with sufficient scientific methods. It is a scientific rather than a legal issue.

Though the UNCLOS allows costal states to deny a foreign ship's right of innocent passage in their territorial waters and prohibit ships from entering for sanitary reasons [17], some ships were actually denied entry into ports without an evidence-based risk assessment (EBRA). The dilemma under the COVID-19 circumstance is that, on the one hand, the EBRA shall be based on actual and existing scientific data and requires professionals to use scientific methods to analyze the relevant data of the coronavirus; on the other hand, the coronavirus as a new disease has a certain degree of concealment in terms of its detection, infection, and transmission, especially at the early stage when not much was known. Therefore, the uncertainty of necessary scientific evidence would lead to hysteresis and insufficiency in applying those rules.

4.1.2. Rescue Obligations of Coastal and Port States

From a legal perspective, when a pandemic outbreak occurs on board and an international cruise ship needs to be rescued, the first thing to ascertain is which country has an obligation to rescue. The UNCLOS stipulates two major types of maritime states: the coastal states and the port states [18]. According to its Article 98, every coastal state shall promote the establishment, operation and maintenance of an adequate and effective search and rescue service regarding safety at sea and where circumstances require cooperation with neighboring states for this purpose. Outbreak of COVID-19 on cruise ships would inevitably endanger passengers and crew members on board as well as the general safety at sea. In this sense, all costal states are under the general obligation of international law to rescue infected ships and people under their jurisdiction.

There are virtually two types of port states: one involves a cruise ship that has already entered the port, and the other involves a scheduled port of call without entering. In the latter case, according to relevant provisions of the IHR [19], if the port of call is an international sanitation port as accredited by the WHO, implying that it has certain sanitary facilities and the necessary capability to take such measures as quarantine on board or ashore, then its state should fulfill the relevant rescue obligations. In addition, the state of the ship's home port shall also undertake the rescue obligation, even in the absence of explicit provisions in existing international conventions and related laws. This is because the home port, as the main place of operation of an international cruise ship, has the closest connection by nature with the ship and therefore should provide assistance to the endangered ship under any circumstance.

4.1.3. The Right of Refusal to Entry

The rescue obligations of coastal and port states have limitations. Under the UNCLOS, the rescue obligation primarily concerns dangerous situations such as typhoons and collisions at sea, under which circumstances the nearby ships are obliged to render assistance when a cruise ship calls for rescue in international waters. The COVID-19 pandemic, whereas, is somewhat different from those circumstances. When a pandemic occurs, not only does the cruise ship require special treatment, but the rescuers, including the port states, also need to consider whether they have the necessary capability to prevent and control infectious disease. This is particularly the case in the early stages of the COVID-19 outbreak when many things were unknown in terms of transmission, containment, and treatment. It would be unjustified to request a costal or port state to undertake rescue obligations while putting its own people at risk. Therefore, in the case of the Westerdam cruise ship, Guam refused to rescue by stating that it had limited resources to "screen, quarantine, or treat 1400 patients at one time", and its "obligation [was] to protect the people of Guam" first [20]. Other ports in Japan, South Korea, Thailand, and the Philippines also denied the ship from entry for similar reasons.

Under UNCLOS, innocent passage through territorial sea is an important right of all ships, as long as it is not prejudicial to the peace, good order, or security of the coastal state [21]. As a balance, the coastal state may take necessary steps in its territorial sea to prevent passage that is not innocent and, in its contiguous zone, may also exercise control necessary to prevent infringement of its custom, immigration or sanitary laws within its territorial sea [22]. Accordingly, the premise of an international cruise ship's innocent passage is not to jeopardize the security of coastal states. In other words, if the coastal state deems that the infected international cruise ship may pose a threat to its own safety, it may choose to deny entry of the ship.

If a ship may bring about serious safety threats, costal states are inclined to refuse its entry. Environmental pollution excuses are mostly seen in the past. For example, in November 2002, when the Greek-operated oil tanker MV Prestige carrying 77,000 tonnes of heavy fuel oil was in danger while passing through the waters near Spain, not only the Spanish but the French and Portuguese governments also refused to allow the ship to dock, as these costal states claimed that such an oil leakage accident would cause tremendous damage to their local ecological environment. Compared with oil pollution, the impact of an unpredictable pandemic could be greater. Hence, it can be assumed that the coastal and port states were under pressure to deny entry of an infected international cruise ship in the COVID-19 pandemic circumstance.

4.2. Who Is Accountable?

Apart from the coastal and port states, there are other stakeholders who are also accountable for the prevention and control of COVID-19 on international cruise ships, we found that the flag state, the cruise ship company, and the states of the nationalities of onboard passengers and crew members are also legally involved.

4.2.1. Flag State

The flag state of an international cruise ship is the jurisdiction under whose laws the ship is registered or licensed, namely, the nationality of the ship. Many international agreements including various IMO conventions require the flag states to effectively exercise their jurisdiction and control in administrative, technical and social matters over ships flying their flags [23]. Hence, when encountering COVID-19 issues, a cruise ship can choose to call at the port of its flag state. Even if the ship is in the waters of other states, its flag state cannot be exempted from those obligations and responsibilities under the flag state principle.

The UNCLOS requires that all ships should have the nationality of the state whose flag they are entitled to fly, and there must be a genuine link between the real owner of the ship and the flag with which the ship flies [24]. However, for various reasons and for a long time, to date there is still no uniform standard in implementing this crucial rule, which has led to the so-called "flag of convenience" problem. According to the UNCTAD's latest Review of Maritime Transport, in 2019, 7 of the world's top 10 ship-owning states had their national flags weight under 20% [25]. Under COVID-19, even though they are legally bound, flag states have neither pressure nor motivation to undertake epidemic prevention and control responsibilities. This is also the underlying reason why most flag states chose to shy away from exercising their jurisdictions when their cruise ships encountered COVID-19 problems.

4.2.2. Cruise Ship Company

While a flag state has the legal authority and responsibility to enforce inspection and safety regulations on international cruise ships that are registered under its flag, the safe operation of ships and the safety of people onboard are primarily the ship operators' responsibility. Article 1 of the IHR defines an operator as "a natural or legal person in charge of a conveyance or their agent," which may include ship operators, ship managers and other enterprises, generally referred to as cruise ship companies. Under the current international law framework, there are regulations that specify responsibilities of the states and cruise ship companies with respect to safety and health issues. Article 24 of the IHR, in particular, provides that a state shall take all practicable measures to ensure that ship operators (a) comply with the health measures recommended by WHO and adopted by the state, (b) inform travelers of the health measures recommended by WHO and adopted by the state for application on board, and (c) permanently keep ships free of sources of infection or contamination, including vectors and reservoirs. Corresponding measures to control sources of infection or contamination may be required to apply if evidence is found. When the COVID-19 pandemic is confirmed as a PHEIC, cruise ship companies are obligated to further strengthen their healthcare measures and to cooperate with authorities of coastal and port states as well as their flag state so as to carry out epidemic prevention and control actions effectively, which includes reporting the ship's actual situation quickly and accurately.

4.2.3. State of Nationality of the People on Board

As far as the protection of human rights is concerned, the states of nationality of passengers and crew members on international cruise ships are also legally accountable when they are in danger during the COVID-19 pandemic. Both international treaties, such as the International Covenant on Economic, Social and Cultural Rights (ICESCR), and national laws contain relevant provisions that require the state of the nationalities of the people on board to protect its citizens, which entails protecting the right to health, i.e., "the highest attainable standards of physical and mental health" [26]. From this perspective, all involved states of nationality are obligated to rescue the infected cruise ship in order to protect their nationals' basic right to health. In the Diamond Princess case, largely out of humanitarianism considerations, Japan eventually decided to permit onboard people to disembark so as to take care of their health. Other states of nationality in this case, such as China and the United States, also arranged to evacuate their nationals and to quarantine them further in their own countries. Indeed, as a UN expert recently pointed out, in the fight against the unprecedented COVID-19 pandemic, binding obligations shall be grounded first and foremost on the right to health framework which compels all parties involved to examine the adequacy of their measures [27].

4.3. Rationality and Legality of Certain Measures

4.3.1. Quarantine at Sea

While the Diamond Princess cruise ship was at berth in the Yokohama Port, the Japanese authorities decided to quarantine the entire ship, including all passengers and crew members, on the sea instead of at a designated medical institution on shore for inspection and observation. Some of the measures brought about challenges in terms of rationality and legality.

According to related international agreements, such as the Convention on the International Regime of Maritimes Ports, the assessing criteria mainly include the necessity, reasonableness, appropriateness, and non-discrimination of applying the measures. Article 28(5) of the IHR provides that, if a suspect or affected ship berths elsewhere than at the port at which the ship was due to berth for reasons beyond the control of the officer in command of the ship, as soon as the competent authority has been informed, it may apply health measures recommended by the WHO or other IHR health measures. Nevertheless, these criteria are generally broad, and, apart from them, there are no other compulsory requirements under existing international legal frameworks. Hence, whether a state's specific measures are legitimate or not, it should be assessed by the applicable laws of the concerned state.

When the Diamond Princess was permitted to berth, Japan as the port state had the discretionary right to take inspection and sanitary measures deemed necessary in accordance with its own domestic laws so as to prevent and control the pandemic, including requiring mandatory quarantine for 14 days. However, the consequence of applying these measures during the quarantine period was that the number of confirmed COVID-19 cases on board continued to rise. There are reasons to doubt that such a situation is directly linked with the quarantine environment of the ship itself as well as certain measures adopted by the Japanese authority. In other words, it appeared that some of Japan's measures failed to fully consider or even ignored whether the cruise ship itself has the necessary conditions for an effective quarantine. If this can be established, then the rationality and appropriateness of these measures adopted on board would be subject to challenge.

4.3.2. Prohibiting Persons on Board from Disembarking

Another controversial measure taken by the Japanese government in the Diamond Princess case was that all passengers and crew members on board were prohibited from disembarking, while some held that those healthy people should be allowed to go on shore first. Article 28(2) of the IHR stipulates that ships "shall not be prevented from embarking or disembarking" for public health reasons. However, again, this may be subject to inspection or other measures necessary to prevent the spread of infection or contamination. Article 43(1) further provides that in response to specific public health risks or PHEIC, a country may apply additional health measures in accordance with its relevant national laws if these measures can achieve the same or a greater level of health protection than WHO recommendations. Such measures shall not be more restrictive of international traffic and not more invasive or intrusive to persons than reasonably available alternatives that would achieve the appropriate level of health protection. In addition, from a human rights perspective, IHR Article 3 requires that "the implementation of these Regulations shall be with full respect for the dignity, human rights and fundamental freedoms of persons". As such, if a country adopts certain public health measures that impose restrictions on free movement or require other interventions at a personal or community level, these measures must consist with human right protection requirements and be balanced with ethical considerations.

In the case of the Diamond Princess, because of the poor circulation of fresh air on board, especially in narrow cabins, being quarantined in such a confined space would be more likely to increase cross-infection. Even for healthy people, their immunity would decrease as a consequence of excessive psychological pressure who suffered from the depressive environment, therefore increasing the probability of infection [28]. In other words, those healthy people quarantined on board are below the appropriate level of health protection and would be more likely to be infected than under normal circumstances. If fact, on the Diamond Princess, it was reported that quarantined passengers and crew members increasingly felt helpless, anxious, and fearful, and over time various degrees of mental and physical exhaustion were common [29]. There are studies showing that close confinement helps the coronavirus to spread on board, and passengers could still infect their room-mates and crew members during cabin quarantine [30]. In this sense, Japan's prohibition of healthy people onboard from disembarking appears problematic.

5. Conclusions

During the COVID-19 pandemic, many international cruise lines were suspended in an effort to prevent the global spread of the new coronavirus disease. Some national governments prohibited foreign cruise ships from entering their ports, making thousands of passengers and seafarers unable to disembark while the ships were at sea. These predicaments highlight the lack of international cooperation and coordination for handling such emergencies. COVID-19 is not the first time that international cruise ships encountered predicaments because of a pandemic. After establishing the public health emergency mechanism under the IHR, the WHO has declared the PHEIC six times. SARS in 2003, the H1N1 influenza in 2013, the Ebola virus disease in 2014, and MERS in 2015 affected the global cruising industry substantially. Similar public health problems are likely to happen again in the future. Therefore, we make the following recommendations for the prevention and control of highly contagious epidemics such as COVID-19 on international cruise ships.

First, it must be recognized that in the era of globalization and in the face of a global pandemic, no single state can manage everything, nor can any single international organization solve the problems independently [31]. The predicaments international cruise ships encountered in the early stages of the COVID-19 pandemic, including the above-mentioned legal controversies, clearly indicate that international coordination and cooperation in this field must be strengthened and improved systemically. For instance, the rapid spread of coronavirus on some cruise ships partially resulted from the design of ships, which prevents the effective inspection and isolation of the disease, and a shortage of quarantine and medical facilities, screening, and monitoring protocols. Therefore, in terms of the technical standards of cruise ships, the international community should jointly revise and upgrade the construction specifications and epidemic prevention standards of cruise ships by means of, inter alia, coordinating expert groups on a ship's air-conditioning systems, ship design, operation, and management, and promoting these more advanced technical standards to key stakeholders via international organizations such as the International Association of Classification Societies (IACS). In the meanwhile, it must be acknowledged that the capabilities of different stakeholders are varied and a national government's priority is always to protect its own citizen's rights. Any future international cooperation shall take into consideration the imbalances among all stakeholders.

Information sharing and management is also crucial for the prevention and control of the pandemic. Operating international cruise lines usually involves multiple ports, states, and regions; in the case of epidemic outbreaks, cruise ship companies are expected to work closely with relevant public health authorities to enforce health requirements. It is particularly necessary for them to collect information on the occurrence and development of the epidemic quickly and accurately and to establish a risk assessment mechanism so as to cope with public health emergencies. In this regard, we advise the port states to consider epidemics as an essential indicator in assessing the safety of cruise ships, make files for each visiting ship, and review their emergency response mechanisms regularly.

All this international cooperation should be rule-based and under the framework of relevant international organizations including the WHO, the IMO, the ILO, and the International Chamber of Shipping (ICS). Their primary mission is to coordinate diversified regulations and practices of different countries, make suggestions on establishing harmonized or even unified rules, and evaluate whether a country is fulfilling its responsibilities and obligations under relevant legal frameworks. In view of the regulatory controversies that occurred during the COVID-19 pandemic, these international organizations are particularly expected to take a leading role in evaluating key international rules embodied in the IHR, the International Labour Convention, the Convention on Facilitation of International Maritime Traffic and the International Convention for the Safety of Life at Sea. We recommend that these organizations be more actively involved in addressing those new legal issues under the COVID-19 pandemic circumstances by way of improving existing cooperation and surveillance mechanisms of involved parties. In view of strengthening the future global health governance framework, a more effective supervisory mechanism is highly recommended so as to harmonize various national laws on pandemic control with the international health standards.

With respect to the specific rules in relation to the prevention and control of COVID-19 on international cruise ships, the future legal frameworks are expected to define more clearly the roles and responsibilities of all stakeholders, especially the coastal states, port authorities, and cruise operators. As a general rule, human rights protection shall be the priority consideration when humanitarian crises occur due to the quarantine of people onboard. Contemporary international law has actually been increasingly highlighting human rights, such as the rights "to just and favourable conditions of work [and] to rest and leisure, including reasonable limitation of working hours and periodic holidays with pay" as stipulated by the UN Human Rights Charter [32]. The general duties to render assistance under the UNCLOS, including requiring coastal states to rescue people whose safety are endangered at sea, are also for humanitarian protection [33]. During the COVID-19 pandemic in 2020, numerous seafarers were stranded on cruise ships and were unable to return home as a result of travel restrictions imposed by various states, leading to a humanitarian and safety crisis [34]. Their fundamental human rights were apparently not well respected and protected. An encouraging move was that, on 8 December 2020, the ILO called for urgent action by adopting a special resolution to address the situation and placed the issue of seafarer's rights at the forefront of state consideration [35]. This is the direction in which the international community shall direct their efforts, and a more explicit highlighting of applicable human rights regulations shall be included in future international health law frameworks.

In line with the human rights principle as well as other UNCLOS rules such as the flag state principle, we recommend further clarification on exercising jurisdiction and distributing responsibilities, so that all involved parties can provide the necessary assistance as much and as conveniently as possible in response to COVID-19 control on international cruise ships. Figure 1 presents the priority order of stakeholders undertaking responsi-bilities. More specifically, when a cruise ship is sailing on international waters that are not within any of the state's jurisdiction, the flag state shall maintain its prior right and obligation to rescue the ship. Other coastal states and states of nationality may exercise jurisdiction on the basis of human rights protection. However, when the ship is on the territorial sea of a coastal state and called at a specific port, we recommend that the port state take precedence so as to implement public health measures in accordance with the IHR and other applicable laws. In the meantime, all other stakeholders of the infected ship, including its flag state, the states of the nationality of those on board, and cruise ship companies, shall also actively coordinate and cooperate to fulfill their responsibilities, respectively. That is, a multiple or combined responsibility mechanism is highly recommended.

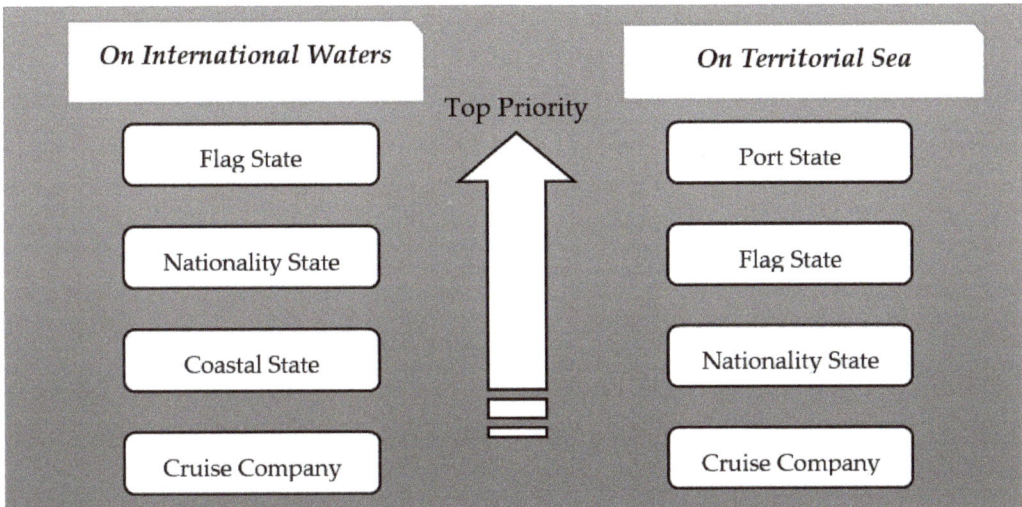

Figure 1. Priority Order of Stakeholders undertaking Responsibilities.

Author Contributions: Conceptualization, C.W. and X.Z.; methodology, X.Z.; formal analysis, C.W. and X.Z.; resources, C.W.; writing—original draft preparation, X.Z.; writing—review and editing, C.W. All authors have read and agreed to the published version of the manuscript.

Funding: This research was funded by China's Social Sciences Foundation "International Legal Issues of the Belt & Road Initiative" (Project No. 15AFX023) and the Academy of International Strategy and Law of Zhejiang University.

Institutional Review Board Statement: Not applicable.

Informed Consent Statement: Not applicable.

Data Availability Statement: The data presented in this study are available on request from the corresponding author.

Acknowledgments: We thank Jinle Ye and Fangmin Ge at The Second Affiliated Hospital of Zhejiang University for their research assistance.

Conflicts of Interest: The authors declare no conflict of interest.

References

1. Statista Research Department. Number of Ocean Cruise Passengers Worldwide from 2009 to 2020. Available online: https://www.statista.com/statistics/385445/number-of-passengers-of-the-cruise-industry-worldwide/ (accessed on 6 November 2020).
2. CNN. Cruise Ship Carrying 8 Passengers Is Last to Dock. Available online: https://edition.cnn.com/travel/article/artania-cruise-ship-docks/index.html (accessed on 6 November 2020).
3. The United States Centers for Disease Control and Prevention. No Sail Order for Cruise Ships. Available online: https://www.cdc.gov/quarantine/cruise/index.html (accessed on 6 November 2020).

4. International Maritime Organization. Crew Changes: A Humanitarian, Safety and Economic Crisis. Available online: https://www.imo.org/en/MediaCentre/HotTopics/Pages/FAQ-on-crew-changes-and-repatriation-of-seafarers.aspx (accessed on 6 November 2020).
5. The United States Centers for Disease Control and Prevention. What CDC Is Doing for Cruise Travelers? Available online: https://www.cdc.gov/coronavirus/2019-ncov/travelers/cruise-ship/what-cdc-is-doing.html (accessed on 6 November 2020).
6. Kate, A.W.; Paul, A.; Jeremy, M.M.; Dwyer, D.E. Outbreaks of pandemic (H1N1) 2009 and seasonal influenza A (H3N2) on cruise ship. *Emerg. Infect. Dis.* **2010**, *16*, 1731–1737. [CrossRef]
7. Cramer, E.H.; Slaten, D.D.; Guerreiro, A.; Robbins, D.; Ganzon, A. Management and control of varicella on cruise ships: A collaborative approach to promoting public health. *J. Travel Med.* **2012**, *19*, 226–232. [CrossRef] [PubMed]
8. BBC. Ruby Princess: New South Wales Premier Apologises over Cruise Ship Outbreak. Available online: https://www.bbc.com/news/world-australia-53802816 (accessed on 16 November 2020).
9. Wikipedia. Available online: https://en.wikipedia.org/wiki/COVID-19_pandemic_on_cruise_ships (accessed on 8 December 2020).
10. World Health Organization. *Handbook for Management of Public Health Events On Board Ships*; World Health Organization: Geneva, Switzerland, 2016; p. 12.
11. International Maritime Organization Resolution, A.949(23), Adopted on 5 December 2003. Available online: https://www.imo.org/en/OurWork/Safety/Pages/PlacesOfRefuge.aspx (accessed on 10 December 2020).
12. International Maritime Organization Resolution, A.950(23), Adopted on 5 December 2003. Available online: https://www.imo.org/en/OurWork/Safety/Pages/PlacesOfRefuge.aspx (accessed on 10 December 2020).
13. Article 28 of the International Health Regulations. 2005. Available online: https://apps.who.int/iris/bitstream/handle/10665/43883/9789241580410_eng.pdf?sequence=1 (accessed on 10 December 2020).
14. Section 3, Subsection A of the United Nations Convention on the Law of the Sea (1982). Available online: https://www.un.org/depts/los/convention_agreements/texts/unclos/unclos_e.pdf (accessed on 12 December 2020).
15. World Health Organization. Director-General's Opening Remarks at the Media Briefing on Ebola and COVID-19 Outbreaks. Available online: https://www.who.int/director-general/speeches/detail/who-director-general-s-opening-remarks-at-the-media-briefing-on-ebola-and-covid-19-outbreaks (accessed on 29 November 2020).
16. Article 43 of the International Health Regulations. 2005. Available online: https://apps.who.int/iris/bitstream/handle/10665/43883/9789241580410_eng.pdf?sequence=1 (accessed on 10 December 2020).
17. Articles 17, 19 and 25 of the United Nations Convention on the Law of the Sea. 1982. Available online: https://www.un.org/depts/los/convention_agreements/texts/unclos/unclos_e.pdf (accessed on 12 December 2020).
18. Erik, M. Port and Coastal States. In *The Oxford Handbook of the Law of the Sea*; Oxford University Press: Oxford, UK, 2015. [CrossRef]
19. Annex 1 of the International Health Regulations. 2005. Available online: https://apps.who.int/iris/bitstream/handle/10665/43883/9789241580410_eng.pdf?sequence=1 (accessed on 10 December 2020).
20. Jerick, S. Guam Denies Entry to Ship over Coronavirus Concerns. Pacific Daily News [7 February 2020]. Available online: https://www.guampdn.com/story/news/local/2020/02/07/guam-denies-entry-ship-over-coronavirus-concerns/4687803002/ (accessed on 16 December 2020).
21. Article 17 and 19 of the United Nations Convention on the Law of the Sea. 1982. Available online: https://www.un.org/depts/los/convention_agreements/texts/unclos/unclos_e.pdf (accessed on 12 December 2020).
22. Article 25 and 33 of the United Nations Convention on the Law of the Sea. 1982. Available online: https://www.un.org/depts/los/convention_agreements/texts/unclos/unclos_e.pdf (accessed on 12 December 2020).
23. Article 5(1) of the Geneva Convention on the High Seas. 1958. Available online: https://www.gc.noaa.gov/documents/8_1_1958_high_seas.pdf (accessed on 12 December 2020).
24. Articles 91, 92 and 94 of the United Nations Convention on the Law of the Sea. 1982. Available online: https://www.un.org/depts/los/convention_agreements/texts/unclos/unclos_e.pdf (accessed on 12 December 2020).
25. The United Nations Conference on Trade and Development. The Review of Maritime Transport. 2019. Available online: https://unctad.org/system/files/official-document/rmt2019_en.pdf (accessed on 16 November 2020).
26. Article 12 of the International Covenant on Economic, Social and Cultural Rights. 1966. Available online: https://www.ohchr.org/EN/ProfessionalInterest/Pages/CESCR.aspx (accessed on 15 December 2020).
27. UN Office of the High Commissioner for Human Rights. COVID-19 measures Must be Grounded First and Foremost on the Right to Health. Available online: https://www.ohchr.org/EN/NewsEvents/Pages/DisplayNews.aspx?NewsID=25945&LangID=E (accessed on 6 December 2020).
28. Battineni, G.; Sagaro, G.G.; Chintalapudi, N.; Di Canio, M.; Amenta, F. Assessment of awareness and knowledge on novel coronavirus (COVID-19) pandemic among seafarers. *Healthcare* **2021**, *9*, 120. [CrossRef] [PubMed]
29. Subramanian, S. The Ordeal of the Diamond Princess Crew. The Diplomat, 22 February 2020. Available online: https://thediplomat.com/2020/02/the-ordeal-of-the-diamond-princess-crew (accessed on 1 December 2020).
30. Smriti, M. What the cruise-ship outbreaks reveal about COVID-19. *Nature* **2020**, *18*, 580. [CrossRef]
31. Luis, A.F.; Antonio, S.; Francisco, S. How will covid-19 impact on the governance of global health in the 2030 agenda framework? The opinion of experts. *Healthcare* **2020**, *8*, 356. [CrossRef]

32. Article 23 and 24 of the Universal Declaration of Human Rights. 1948. Available online: https://www.un.org/en/universal-declaration-human-rights/ (accessed on 12 December 2020).
33. Article 98 of the United Nations Convention on the Law of the Sea. 1982. Available online: https://www.un.org/depts/los/convention_agreements/texts/unclos/unclos_e.pdf (accessed on 12 December 2020).
34. International Maritime Organization. A humanitarian Crisis at Sea: All United Nations Member States Must Resolve the Crew Change Crisis [14 September 2020]. Available online: https://www.imo.org/en/MediaCentre/PressBriefings/Pages/27-crew-change-joint-statement.aspx (accessed on 26 December 2020).
35. International Labour Organization. Resolution Concerning Maritime Labour Issues and the Covid-19 Pandemic, Adopted on the 340th Session of the Governing Body of the ILO [8 December 2020]. Available online: https://www.ilo.org/gb/GBSessions/GB340/WCMS_760649/lang--en/index.htm (accessed on 26 December 2020).

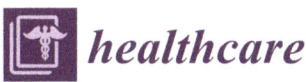 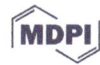

Article

Predictors of Staying at Home during the COVID-19 Pandemic and Social Lockdown based on Protection Motivation Theory: A Cross-Sectional Study in Japan

Tsuyoshi Okuhara *, Hiroko Okada and Takahiro Kiuchi

Department of Health Communication, School of Public Health, The University of Tokyo, Tokyo 113-8655, Japan; okadahiroko-tky@umin.ac.jp (H.O.); tak-kiuchi@umin.ac.jp (T.K.)
* Correspondence: okuhara-ctr@umin.ac.jp; Tel.: +81-3-5800-6549

Received: 30 September 2020; Accepted: 7 November 2020; Published: 11 November 2020

Abstract: During the COVID-19 pandemic, a social lockdown should be put in place and individuals should stay at home. Behavioral change is the only way to prevent the pandemic and overwhelmed healthcare systems until vaccines are available. We aimed to examine the psychological factors that predict staying at home during the COVID-19 pandemic and social lockdown. A total of 1980 participants in Japan completed a survey for this study from 9 to 11 May 2020, when the state of emergency covered all prefectures in the country. Self-reported behavior in terms of staying at home, the perceived severity of the pandemic, vulnerability to the pandemic, response efficacy, and self-efficacy based on protection motivation theory were assessed. Multiple regression analysis showed that perceived severity (standardized $\beta = 0.11$, $p < 0.001$) and self-efficacy (standardized $\beta = 0.32$, $p < 0.001$) significantly predicted greater levels of staying at home, after controlling for socio-demographics. However, perceived vulnerability and response efficacy did not. To encourage people to stay at home during the pandemic and social lockdown, increasing the perceived severity of infection by COVID-19 and self-efficacy in terms of exercising restraint with respect to going out may consequently encourage people to stay at home.

Keywords: COVID-19; novel coronavirus; social lockdown; protection motivation theory; health behavior; health communication

1. Introduction

The outbreak of the coronavirus disease (COVID-19) has emerged as the largest global pandemic in recent history [1]. Currently, no medicine has been identified for the treatment of the disease [2]. COVID-19 is a transmissible disease that can be passed from an infected individual through any object that carries the virus to anyone who comes into contact with it. Therefore, social lockdown has been recommended by health experts as a preventive measure [3,4]. Social lockdown is a restriction of inter-individual physical contacts [5]. Under social lockdown, unnecessary movements and contacts between individuals are not allowed. Experts have proposed that social lockdown would generate better consequences, such as controlling the increase in the number of infected individuals, restricting community infection, preventing the healthcare system from becoming overloaded, and providing better health care to the infected individuals [5]. Owing to its importance, the governments of many countries across the world have declared local and national social lockdowns [5,6].

In Japan, the government declared a state of emergency on 7 April 2020 [7]. The state of emergency allowed the prefectural governors to request residents to refrain from unnecessary and non-urgent outings, and also to request business operators to restrict their use of stores and facilities [7]. Initially, the state of emergency covered the period from 8 April 2020 to 6 May 2020, and the target area was seven prefectures, including Tokyo and Osaka [7]. As of 7 April 2020, the number of infected individuals was 4625, and the number of deaths was 80 [8]. Those numbers rapidly increased after the declaration, rising to 14,034 cases and 170 deaths as of 15 April 2020 [8]. Therefore, on 16 April 2020, the area covered by the state of emergency was expanded to all prefectures in Japan [9]. Moreover, the Japanese government designated "specified warning prefectures" where there had been a particular increase in the number of infected individuals. There were six "specified warning prefectures", including Hokkaido and Kyoto, in addition to the seven prefectures targeted first [9]. Furthermore, on 2 May 2020, the target period was extended to 31 May 2020 [9].

However, the Japanese state of emergency had few legally enforceable measures [10], and it was not a legal lockdown of the type imposed in some countries [11]. The Japanese stay-at-home order was just a "request" by the governors, and they had no legal powers to penalize individuals who disregarded calls to stay at home [11]. Accordingly, only about 40% of individuals reduced their frequency of shopping trips, and only about 30% reduced outing for the purpose of commuting in the seven prefectures first targeted in the state of emergency between a week and ten days after the declaration of emergency [12]. Even in countries in Europe and states in the U.S. where the lockdown had legal force, some people resisted it and disregarded calls to stay at home (e.g., [13,14]). Even if the number of newly infected individuals decreases, relaxing the interventions and resuming going out could cause a second wave of the spread of infections [15]. Because social lockdown is the only existing weapon to prevent the spread of the COVID-19 pandemic until vaccines are available to halt it, changing individuals' behavior regarding staying at home is crucial [5].

In the early stages of a pandemic, effective communication of risk and preventive behaviors to the general public is one of the main public health strategies to reduce morbidity and mortality [16–19]. Protection motivation theory (PMT) [20,21] is one of the behavioral change theories that have been employed in such public health communications during pandemics [22,23]. PMT assumes that the motivation (i.e., intention) to protect oneself from danger is determined by two processes: threat appraisal and coping appraisal. Threat appraisal depends on the perceived severity of the health threat and on the perceived vulnerability to it. Coping appraisal depends on the perceived response efficacy (i.e., evaluation of whether the behavior is effective for alleviating the threat) and on perceived self-efficacy (i.e., evaluation of whether one will be able to carry out the behavior). PMT posits a positive linear relationship between the threat and coping appraisals and behavioral intention. In fact, previous studies showed that individuals' perceived severity of the situation, vulnerability to the situation, response efficacy, and self-efficacy predicted their motivation to protect themselves during an influenza pandemic [22–25].

It is crucial to investigate factors that predict the behavior of staying at home during the COVID-19 pandemic, especially psychological factors that can be influenced through interventions. One previous study investigated the impact of online information regarding the intention to voluntarily self-isolate during the pandemic in Finland using PMT as a framework [26]. That study reported that perceived severity and self-efficacy had a positive impact on self-isolation intention [26]. However, no studies have investigated the relationship between PMT constructs and the intention to stay at home in Japan. Such an investigation is urgent under the situation where the Japanese state of emergency only included a few legally enforceable measures, as mentioned earlier. If psychological factors that predict the behavior of staying at home during the COVID-19 pandemic are revealed, the findings will contribute to more persuasive public health campaigns to encourage people to stay at home in Japan. Such public health campaigns are especially important in situations where vaccines are not yet available. We aimed to examine the psychological factors that predict the behavior of staying at home during the COVID-19 pandemic and social lockdown based on the PMT. Our research question was which construct of PMT predicted staying at home during the COVID-19 pandemic and social lockdown in Japan.

2. Materials and Methods

2.1. Study Design and Setting

This cross-sectional study was conducted from 9 May 2020 to 11 May 2020, when the state of emergency covered all prefectures in Japan. This cross-sectional study was conducted as part of another intervention study in Japan [27]. Participants in this cross-sectional study were the same as those in that intervention study. The sample size was determined for that intervention study [27]. Based on the effect size in a previous randomized controlled study [28], we estimated a small effect size (Cohen's d = 0.20) in that intervention study [27]. We conducted a power analysis at an alpha error rate of 0.05 (two-tailed) and a beta error rate of 0.20. The power analysis indicated that 330 participants were required in each of the five intervention groups and one control group (i.e., 1980 participants in total). All participants in this study responded to all measures described below prior to the intervention in that study.

2.2. Participants and Procedures

The participants were recruited from people registered in a survey company database in Japan. E-mails were sent to 47,874 registered users. Of those, 5599 e-mail recipients responded to screening questions. Men and women aged 18–69 years were eligible to participate. The exclusion criteria were individuals who answered in the affirmative to screening questions asking if they are unable to cooperate with a study on the novel coronavirus infection being conducted by the University of Tokyo; if they could not go out due to illness or disability; if they had been diagnosed with a mental illness; or if they or their family members had been infected with COVID-19. In total, 1320 individuals were excluded from the screening questions.

A total of 4279 respondents who were determined to be eligible and consented to participate were invited to complete a web-based survey. The respondents answered questions on a computer or smartphone that was connected to the Internet. We stopped the invitations to complete the web-based survey once 3569 individuals had completed the survey. We set the number to 3569 individuals so as to recruit a larger sample of respondents than the required sample size, to avoid under-sampling owing to incomplete responses. A database of the survey company was used for allocation of sex, age, and residential area. Finally, 1980 participants were randomly selected from among the 3569 respondents. That random selection was conducted in keeping with the allocation according to the population composition ratio of Japan.

2.3. Ethical Considerations

The protocol was approved by the ethical review committee at the Graduate School of Medicine, University of Tokyo (number 2020032NI). All participants gave written informed consent in accordance with the Declaration of Helsinki.

2.4. Measures

2.4.1. Sociodemographic Measures

The participants were asked for their sociodemographic information: gender, age, residential prefecture, educational background, and household income.

2.4.2. Dependent Variable

Because there was no validated scale to assess behaviors of staying at home that was applicable to the present study, a measure was adapted from previous studies of influenza pandemic [29,30] and modified. Namely, from those measures of the previous studies [29,30], we excluded a question about the reduction of the amount of using public transport because those who live in city areas use public transport whereas those who live in rural areas use cars in Japan. We also excluded a question about taking time off work because it depended on workplaces whether to allow workers to commute to work under the Japanese state of emergency. Additionally, we changed a term of "the new flu" in the measures of those previous studies [29,30] to "the novel coronavirus" in the present study. In the present study, the participants responded to the following three questions on 1–10 scales ranging from "same as normal" to "not going out at all": (1) Have you deliberately canceled or postponed plans such as "meeting people," "eating out," or "attending events" because of the novel coronavirus infection? (2) Have you deliberately reduced the time you spend shopping in stores outside your home because of the novel coronavirus infection? (3) Have you deliberately avoided crowded spaces because of the novel coronavirus infection? A mean score was calculated.

2.4.3. Independent Variables

For perceived severity, the participants responded to the following two questions: (1) How seriously do you think your health will be affected if you are infected with the novel coronavirus? (2) How serious do you think the social situation will be if the novel coronavirus spreads? For perceived vulnerability, participants responded to the following two questions: (1) How likely are you to be infected with the novel coronavirus? (2) How likely are you to be infected with the novel coronavirus when compared to someone of the same sex and age as you? These measures were adapted from previous studies [31,32]. We changed a term of "the new flu" in the measures of those previous studies [31,32] to "the novel coronavirus" in the present study. For perceived response efficacy, participants responded to the following explanation and three questions: Please share your thoughts on the effectiveness of staying at home to prevent the spread of novel coronavirus infection. (1) Do you think that you can save your life from the new coronavirus infection and prevent the spread of infection by canceling or postponing appointments such as "meeting people," "eating out," and "attending events"? (2) . . . . by reducing the time you spend shopping at stores outside your home? (3) . . . . by avoiding crowded spaces? For perceived self-efficacy, participants responded to the following explanation and three questions: Please share your thoughts regarding your confidence in the effectiveness of staying at home to prevent the spread of novel coronavirus infections. (1) Do you think that you can cancel or postpone appointments such as "meeting people," "eating out," and "attending events" because of the novel coronavirus infection? (2) Do you think you can reduce the time you spend shopping in stores outside your home . . . .? (3) Do you think you can avoid crowded spaces . . . .? Because there was no validated scale to assess response efficacy and self-efficacy regarding the COVID-19 pandemic, these measures were adapted from previous studies [29,30]. We changed a term of "the new flu" in the measures of those previous studies [29,30] to "the novel coronavirus" in the present study. The participants responded to these questions based on PMT on 1–6 scales on which the intervals indicated "extremely unlikely," "unlikely," "a little unlikely," "a little likely," "likely," or "extremely likely" in ascending order. Mean scores were calculated for these measures. Higher scores indicated greater intention and perception.

2.5. Statistical Analysis

Cronbach's α values were used to determine internal reliability of the measures. Descriptive statistics were used to describe participants' sociodemographic information by summarizing categorical variables in percentage terms and giving mean ± SD for continuous variables. The residential areas of the participants were dichotomized to a binary variable indicating whether or not the area was within the "specified warning prefectures". We examined the associations between sociodemographic information and staying at home using a two-sample t-test and a one-way ANOVA. We then calculated Pearson's product-moment correlations to examine the simple association among study variables. We employed multiple regression analysis using perceived severity, vulnerability, response efficacy, self-efficacy, and sociodemographic measures as independent variables, and staying at home as a dependent variable. Additionally, we conducted subgroup analyses including only participants who lived in the "specified warning prefectures" using multiple regression analysis. In those multiple regression analyses, sociodemographic measures such as sex, age, educational background, and household income were included, based on published literature [16,23]. Participants' residential area and whether they were living in one of the specified warning prefectures were also used as independent variables because they were presumed to be related to participants' social behavior and social lockdown in Japan during the COVID-19 pandemic. A p-value of < 0.05 was set as significant in all statistical tests. All statistical analyses were performed using IBM SPSS Statistics for Windows, Version 21.0 (IBM Corp., Armonk, NY, USA).

3. Results

3.1. Descriptive Statistics

The mean values of the participants' responses to the questions about staying at home were as follows: 7.25 (SD = 2.51) for canceling or postponing plans; 6.39 (SD = 2.51) for a reduction in time spent shopping; 7.67 (SD = 2.17) for the avoidance of crowded spaces. The Cronbach's α values for the internal consistency of the responses to the questions were as follows: 0.835 for the behavior of staying at home; 0.480 for perceived severity; 0.875 for vulnerability; 0.921 for response efficacy; 0.853 for self-efficacy. Table 1 shows the participants' characteristics and their associations with staying at home. As mentioned earlier, the participants' sex, age, and place of residence were consistent with the population composition ratio in Japan. The behavior of staying at home was significantly associated with gender ($p < 0.001$), younger age ($p = 0.002$), residential area ($p < 0.001$), being in one of the specified warning prefectures ($p < 0.001$), higher educational background ($p < 0.001$), and larger household income ($p < 0.001$).

Table 1. Sociodemographic characteristics of the participants and their associations with staying at home ($n = 1980$).

Sociodemographic Characteristics	Overall (%)	Mean (SD) [a]	p
Gender			
Men	49.7	6.76 (2.2)	<0.001 [b]
Women	50.3	7.45 (1.9)	
Age			
18–29 years old	16.1	7.39 (1.9)	0.002 [c]
Men	50.9		
30–39 years old	18.5	7.32 (2.0)	
Men	50.8		
40–49 years old	23.6	7.03 (2.2)	
Men	50.0		
50–59 years old	20.6	7.00 (2.1)	
Men	50.0		
60–69 years old	21.2	6.88 (2.2)	
Men	47.1		
Residential area			
Hokkaido	4.8	7.10 (2.2)	<0.001 [c]
Tohoku	7.9	6.46 (2.3)	
Kanto	32.4	7.37 (1.9)	
Hokuriku and Chubu	17.9	6.89 (2.3)	
Kinki	16.7	7.22 (1.9)	
Chugoku and Shikoku	8.8	6.75 (2.3)	
Kyushu and Okinawa	11.5	7.22 (1.9)	
Specified warning prefectures			
Applicable	64.3	7.31 (1.9)	<0.001 [b]
Not applicable	35.7	6.73 (2.3)	

Table 1. Cont.

Sociodemographic Characteristics	Overall (%)	Mean (SD) [a]	p
Highest education			
Less than high school	1.7	6.40 (2.5)	<0.001 [c]
High school graduate	26.0	6.79 (2.3)	
Some college	24.1	7.12 (2.2)	
College graduate	40.7	7.27 (1.9)	
Graduate school	7.5	7.40 (1.5)	
Household income [d]			
Less than 2 million yen	9.2	6.57 (2.6)	<0.001 [c]
2–6 million yen	43.9	7.07 (2.1)	
More than 6 million yen	37.2	7.34 (1.7)	
Unknown	9.6	6.87 (2.4)	

[a] Standard deviation. [b] two-sample t-test. [c] a one-way ANOVA. [d] One US dollar is roughly equivalent to 100 yen.

Table 2 shows the bivariate intercorrelations among study variables. Perceived severity, response efficacy, and self-efficacy showed positive correlations with staying at home and gender with weak to moderate associations ($p < 0.001$), respectively. However, perceived vulnerability did not. Perceived severity showed weak positive correlations with greater age, perceived vulnerability, response efficacy, and self-efficacy ($p < 0.001$, respectively). Perceived response efficacy showed a moderate positive correlation with self-efficacy ($p < 0.001$).

Table 2. Correlations between variables (n = 1980).

.	Mean (SD)	1.	2.	3.	4.	5.	6.	7.	8.	9.
1. Staying at home	7.10 (2.08)									
2. Gender [a]	-	0.17 **								
3. Age	-	−0.09 **	0.01							
4. Specified warning prefectures [b]	-	0.13**	0.02	−0.01						
5. Education	-	0.11 **	−0.20 **	−0.18 **	0.13 **					
6. Income	-	0.06 *	−0.03	0.01	0.03	0.12 **	−0.01			
7. Severity	4.33 (0.86)	0.18 **	0.07 **	0.12 **	−0.03	−0.07 **	−0.01			
8. Vulnerability	3.10 (0.91)	0.03	0.02	−0.08 **	0.03	0.02	0.02	0.26 **		
9. Response efficacy	4.44 (0.82)	0.29 **	0.13 **	−0.03	0.03	−0.01	0.03	0.23 **	−0.04 *	
10. Self-efficacy	4.68 (0.75)	0.39 **	0.15 **	−0.00	0.05*	−0.03	0.03	0.23 **	−0.03	0.64 **

* $p < 0.05$; ** $p < 0.001$. [a] The reference category is men. [b] The reference category is prefectures other than the specified warning prefectures.

3.2. Regression Analysis

As shown in Table 3, when including all prefectures, perceived severity (Standardized β = 0.11, $p < 0.001$) and self-efficacy (Standardized β = 0.32, $p < 0.001$) significantly predicted more staying at home, controlling for gender, age, residential area, being in one of the specified warning prefectures, educational background, and household income. However, perceived vulnerability and response efficacy did not. The independent variables explained 21% of the variance in the dependent variable (adjusted $R^2 = 0.21$).

The number of participants who lived in the "specified warning prefectures" was 1274. When including only participants who lived in the "specified warning prefectures", perceived severity (Standardized β = 0.07, $p = 0.006$) and self-efficacy (Standardized β = 0.342, $p < 0.001$) significantly predicted more staying at home. However, perceived vulnerability and response efficacy did not.

Table 3. Regression analysis to predict staying at home ($n = 1980$) (Adjusted $R^2 = 0.21$).

Variables	β	SE	95% CI	Std β	t	p
(Intercept)	−0.25	0.45	[−1.13, 0.63]		−0.55	0.580
Gender [a]	0.54	0.09	[0.37, 0.71]	0.13	6.29	0.000
Age	−0.01	0.00	[−0.02, −0.01]	−0.09	−4.13	0.000
Residential area	0.04	0.03	[−0.01, 0.09]	0.03	1.49	0.137
Specified warning prefectures [b]	0.47	0.09	[0.29, 0.64]	0.11	5.14	0.000
Education	0.25	0.05	[0.16, 0.33]	0.12	5.49	0.000
Income	0.10	0.05	[−0.01, 0.20]	0.04	1.81	0.070
Severity	0.27	0.05	[0.16, 0.37]	0.11	5.03	0.000
Vulnerability	−0.02	0.05	[−0.11, 0.08]	−0.01	−0.32	0.746
Response efficacy	0.10	0.07	[−0.03, 0.23]	0.04	1.46	0.145
Self-efficacy	0.88	0.07	[0.74, 1.02]	0.32	12.10	0.000

SE = Standard Error. CI = Confidence Interval [lower-bound, upper-bound]. Std β = Standardized β. [a] The reference category is men. [b] The reference category is prefectures other than the specified warning prefectures.

4. Discussion

The regression analysis in the present study found that, of the four variables in the PMT, perceived severity and self-efficacy were significant predictors of staying at home during the COVID-19 pandemic and social lockdown in all Japanese prefectures, as well as the "specified warning prefectures". This result was consistent with a previous study of voluntary self-isolation based on the PMT conducted during the COVID-19 pandemic in Finland, in which perceived severity and self-efficacy positively impacted self-isolation intention [26]. Perceived self-efficacy was a stronger predictor than perceived severity in the present study. This finding was consistent with previous studies of preventive behavior in the context of pandemic influenza, which showed that perceived self-efficacy is the strongest predictor of the intention of staying at home among the variables in the PMT [24,25]. These studies of pandemic influenza also showed that perceived severity was a significant predictor of staying at home [24,25], as found in this study.

However, perceived vulnerability and response efficacy were not significant predictors of staying at home in this study. This finding was inconsistent with previous studies [24,25]. As Table 2 shows, the perceived vulnerability of the participants in this study was not high: the mean value was 3.10, and participants' response of 3 on a 1–6 scale was equivalent to a perception of being "a little unlikely" to be infected. This indicates that the participants in this study thought that they were unlikely to be infected and, therefore, that they were not motivated to restrain themselves from going out. Communication to increase perceived vulnerability is thus necessary. For example, health professionals and the mass media should place more emphasis on the fact that a characteristic of the novel coronavirus is that it is sometimes difficult to notice that someone is infected and, consequently, that it is hard to prevent infection if people come into contact with others. On the contrary, as Table 2 shows, the perceived response efficacy of the participants in this study was not low (mean = 4.44). This indicates that, even if the participants in this study thought that staying at home was somewhat effective in saving their lives and the spread of the disease, they were not motivated to restrain themselves from going out. This inference may indicate the difficulty of voluntary self-restraint with respect to going out.

The results of this study indicate that perceived severity rather than vulnerability should be increased to increase the threat appraisal, and that perceived self-efficacy rather than response efficacy should be improved to increase the coping appraisal, in order to encourage staying at home during the COVID-19 pandemic and social lockdown in Japan. To increase the perceived severity of infection with COVID-19, narrative communication can be a tool [33,34], e.g., a narrative message from a patient that conveys how severe the consequences of COVID-19 are [35]. Another example is a narrative message from a physician, stating that no treatment is available for COVID-19, that some patients rapidly develop severe symptoms, and that hospitals are overwhelmed [36]. Although social lockdown presumably evoked psychological reactance in many individuals [37], studies indicated that narrative messages obfuscate persuasive intent, subsequently reducing the psychological reactance and generating more persuasiveness than expository messages [38–40].

The heuristic rule of social norms—how others act in a given situation—is the self-protection system acquired by humans throughout evolutionary history [41] and has been shown to influence individuals' judgment and behaviors [42]. In particular, it has been proposed that Japanese individuals has a collectivistic culture, and that there is a lot of pressure to conform to others in Japan [43]. Japanese individuals tend to be susceptible and influenced by information about how others act in a given situation [43]. Therefore, the heuristic rule of social norms can be used to increase perceived self-efficacy to stay at home [44]. For example, messages such as indicating the rate of reduction of movement of people, showing a picture of a downtown location without any people, and communicating narratives of people who spend time meaningfully at home, may increase self-efficacy to stay at home [44,45]. Additionally, providing behavioral alternatives, such as amusements at home or online social interaction, can also be a strategy to reduce psychological reactance and increase self-efficacy [46,47]. Public health experts, physicians and nurses, media workers, and individuals in general may be able to increase perceived severity and self-efficacy and subsequently encourage people to stay at home by disseminating such messages through the mass media and social networking services on the internet. Further, exposure to images of illness and death and news that inspires fear can increase anxiety and decrease confidence in coping with pandemic. Therefore, to avoid bias in news coverage, it will be crucial that public health professionals to work more effectively with the media; e.g., being readily accessible for journalists and providing reliable and useful information resources [48].

Finally, multiple regression analysis in this study found that female gender, younger age, and higher educational background were associated with more staying at home. The gender difference in this study was consistent with previous studies that females engaged in more precautionary behavior than their male counterparts during a swine flu pandemic [29,49] and pandemic COVID-19 [50], and with a literature review that indicated that females more often reported higher levels of risk as a concern than do males in general [51]. There has been discussion of social roles as a possible cause: due to their role as nurturer and care provider, females tend to avoid risks more than males, and due to their role as income earner, males tend to avoid risks less than females [51]. The reason why younger participants tended to stay at home may have been that they had more choices of home entertainment using the internet than older participants [52]. A higher educational background may contribute to the formation of enduring cognitive and emotional skills to foster health decisions, such as adopting behaviors to protect oneself against infectious diseases [53]. These results also should be considered for future research and practice to encourage people stay at home during pandemic.

Our study has several limitations. While the use of a panel database and a web-based survey had the advantage of allowing us to quickly recruit participants under the state of emergency, the selection bias of participants needs to be taken into account when interpreting the study results; participants in the present study did not represent the Japanese population. We assessed self-reported behavior rather than objectively measured behavior. The study results should be interpreted with caution because the measures used in the present study have not been validated and outcome scores may not appropriately reflect participants' perception and behavior. The independent variables in this study did not include the response costs, as in some previous studies of infectious disease using PMT [54,55]. The cross-sectional design of this study constrains the ability to make causal inferences. Longitudinal research and randomized controlled studies will be necessary in the future to examine the temporal, causal relations. It is unclear to what extent the present findings are generalizable to populations other than the participants in this study.

5. Conclusions

During the COVID-19 pandemic and social lockdown in Japan, perceived severity and self-efficacy were the significant predictors of staying at home among the variables of the PMT. Perceived self-efficacy was a stronger predictor than perceived severity. Our findings indicate that, when encouraging people to stay at home during a pandemic, increasing perceived severity and self-efficacy by public health campaigns may consequently encourage people to stay at home. In future research, intervention studies will be needed to examine persuasive message content in terms of psychological factors, to encourage people to stay at home, e.g., determining whether intervention messages that increase perceived severity and self-efficacy encourage recipients to stay at home. We call for more studies to examine psychological factors that can encourage people to stay at home, especially in countries hit by second and third waves of infection. Public health experts, physicians and nurses, media workers, and influential individuals should disseminate messages that have been verified as influential by such studies. In that way, public health research, campaigns, and subsequent changes in individual behavior can help to slow the COVID-19 pandemic. Furthermore, examining psychological factors and messages to encourage people to stay at home based on the behavioral change theories will contribute to prevent the spread of other highly infectious diseases in the future as well.

Author Contributions: Conceptualization, T.O. and H.O.; methodology, T.O. and H.O.; investigation, T.O. and H.O.; formal analysis, T.O.; original draft preparation, T.O.; writing—review and editing, T.O., H.O. and T.K.; supervision, T.K.; funding acquisition, T.O. All authors have read and agreed to the published version of the manuscript.

Funding: This research was supported by a Japan Society for the Promotion of Science KAKENHI [grant number 19K10615].

Conflicts of Interest: The authors declare no conflict of interest.

References

1. World Health Organization. Coronavirus Disease (COVID-19) Pandemic. 2020. Available online: https://www.who.int/emergencies/diseases/novel-coronavirus-2019 (accessed on 15 May 2020).
2. U.S. Food and Drug Administration. FDA COVID-19 Response. In *At-A-Glance Summary*; U.S. Food and Drug Administration: Silver Spring, MD, USA, 14 April 2020.
3. Lau, H.; Khosrawipour, V.; Kocbach, P.; Mikolajczyk, A.; Schubert, J.; Bania, J.; Khosrawipour, T. The positive impact of lockdown in Wuhan on containing the COVID-19 outbreak in China. *J. Travel Med.* **2020**, *27*, taaa037. [CrossRef] [PubMed]
4. Iacobucci, G. Covid-19: UK lockdown is "crucial" to saving lives, say doctors and scientists. *BMJ* **2020**, *368*, m1204. [CrossRef] [PubMed]
5. Paital, B.; Das, K.; Parida, S.K. Inter nation social lockdown versus medical care against COVID-19, a mild environmental insight with special reference to India. *Sci. Total Environ.* **2020**, *728*, 138914. [CrossRef] [PubMed]
6. BBC News. Coronavirus: The World in Lockdown in Maps and Charts. Available online: https://www.bbc.com/news/world-52103747 (accessed on 15 May 2020).
7. The Ministry of Health, Labour and Welfare. Available online: https://www.jda.or.jp/dentist/coronavirus/upd/file/20200413_coronavirus_kinkyujitaisengen_kihontekitaisyohousin49.pdf (accessed on 15 May 2020).
8. COVID-19 Japan Case by Each Prefecture. Available online: https://gis.jag-japan.com/covid19jp/ (accessed on 15 May 2020).
9. The Ministry of Health, Labour and Welfare. Available online: https://corona.go.jp/news/pdf/kinkyujitaisengen_gaiyou0416.pdf (accessed on 15 May 2020).
10. Office for Novel Coronavirus Disease Control, Cabinet Secretariat, Government of Japan. 2020. Available online: https://corona.go.jp/news/news_20200411_53.html (accessed on 15 May 2020).
11. NHK. Available online: https://www3.nhk.or.jp/news/special/coronavirus/tokyo/emergency.html (accessed on 15 May 2020).
12. Yahoo! Japan News, What Outings Have been Reduced by the Declaration of a State of Emergency Against the Novel Coronavirus, and to What Extent? Available online: https://news.yahoo.co.jp/byline/hiroiu/20200419-00174187/ (accessed on 15 May 2020).

13. BBC News, Coronavirus: The US Resistance to a Continued Lockdown. Available online: https://www.bbc.com/news/world-us-canada-52417610 (accessed on 15 May 2020).
14. REUTERS, "I Want my Life Back": Germans Protest Against Lockdown. Available online: https://jp.reuters.com/article/us-health-coronavirus-germany-protests/i-want-my-life-back-germans-protest-against-lockdown-idUKKCN2270RD (accessed on 15 May 2020).
15. Xu, S.; Li, Y. Beware of the second wave of COVID-19. *Lancet* **2020**, *395*, 1321–1322. [CrossRef]
16. Lin, L.; Savoia, E.; Agboola, F.; Viswanath, K. What have we learned about communication inequalities during the H1N1 pandemic: A systematic review of the literature. *BMC Public Health* **2014**, *14*, 484. [CrossRef] [PubMed]
17. Finset, A.; Bosworth, H.; Butow, P.; Gulbrandsen, P.; Hulsman, R.L.; Pieterse, A.H.; Street, R.; Tschoetschel, R.; van Weert, J. Effective health communication—A key factor in fighting the COVID-19 pandemic. *Patient Educ. Couns.* **2020**, *103*, 873–876. [CrossRef]
18. Risk Communication and Community Engagement (RCCE). Action Plan Guidance COVID-19 Preparedness and Response. Available online: https://www.who.int/publications-detail/risk-communication-and-community-engagement-(rcce)-action-plan-guidance (accessed on 1 November 2020).
19. Lunn, P.D.; Belton, C.A.; Lavin, C.; McGowan, F.P.; Timmons, S.; Robertson, D.A. Using Behavioural Science to Help Fight the Coronavirus. 2020. Available online: https://www.esri.ie/publications/using-behavioural-science-to-help-fight-the-coronavirus (accessed on 1 November 2020).
20. Rogers, R.D. A protection motivation theory. *J. Psychol.* **1975**, *91*, 93–114. [CrossRef]
21. Maddux, J.E.; Rogers, R.W. Protection motivation and self-efficacy: A revised theory of fear appeals and attitude change. *J. Exp. Soc. Psychol.* **1983**, *19*, 469–479. [CrossRef]
22. Bish, A.; Yardley, L.; Nicoll, A.; Michie, S. Factors associated with uptake of vaccination against pandemic influenza: A systematic review. *Vaccine* **2011**, *29*, 6472–6484. [CrossRef]
23. Bish, A.; Michie, S. Demographic and attitudinal determinants of protective behaviours during a pandemic: A review. *Br. J. Health Psychol.* **2010**, *15*, 797–824. [CrossRef]
24. Teasdale, E.; Yardley, L.; Schlotz, W.; Michie, S. The importance of coping appraisal in behavioural responses to pandemic flu. *Br. J. Health Psychol.* **2012**, *17*, 44–59. [CrossRef] [PubMed]
25. Timpka, T.; Spreco, A.; Gursky, E.; Eriksson, O.; Dahlström, Ö.; Strömgren, M.; Ekberg, J.; Pilemalm, S.; Karlsson, D.; Hinkula, J.; et al. Intentions to perform non-pharmaceutical protective behaviors during influenza outbreaks in Sweden: A cross-sectional study following a mass vaccination campaign. *PLoS ONE* **2014**, *9*, e91060. [CrossRef] [PubMed]
26. Farooq, A.; Laato, S.; Najmul Islam, A.K.M. Impact of online information self-isolation intention during the COVID-19 Pandemic: Cross-Sectional study. *J. Med. Internet Res.* **2020**, *22*, 1–15. [CrossRef] [PubMed]
27. Okuhara, T.; Okada, H.; Kiuchi, T. Examining persuasive message type to encourage staying at home during the COVID-19 pandemic and social lockdown: A randomized controlled study in Japan. *Patient Educ. Couns.* **2020**. [CrossRef]
28. Hopfer, S. Effects of a Narrative HPV Vaccination Intervention Aimed at Reaching College Women: A Randomized Controlled Trial. *Prev. Sci.* **2012**, *13*, 173–182. [CrossRef]
29. Rubin, G.J.; Amlôt, R.; Page, L.; Wessely, S. Public perceptions, anxiety, and behaviour change in relation to the swine flu outbreak: Cross sectional telephone survey. *BMJ* **2009**, *339*, 156. [CrossRef]
30. Bults, M.; Beaujean, D.J.M.A.; De Zwart, O.; Kok, G.; Van Empelen, P.; Van Steenbergen, J.E.; Richardus, J.H.; Voeten, H.A.C.M. Perceived risk, anxiety, and behavioural responses of the general public during the early phase of the Influenza A (H1N1) pandemic in the Netherlands: Results of three consecutive online surveys. *BMC Public Health* **2011**, *11*, 2. [CrossRef]
31. Renner, B.; Reuter, T. Predicting vaccination using numerical and affective risk perceptions: The case of A/H1N1 influenza. *Vaccine* **2012**, *30*, 7019–7026. [CrossRef]
32. Reuter, T.; Renner, B. Who takes precautionary action in the face of the new H1N1 influenza? Prediction of who collects a free hand sanitizer using a health behavior model. *PLoS ONE* **2011**, *6*, e22130. [CrossRef]
33. Shelby, A.; Ernst, K. Story and science: How providers and parents can utilize storytelling to combat anti-vaccine misinformation. *Hum. Vaccines Immunother.* **2013**, *9*, 1795–1801. [CrossRef]
34. Hinyard, L.J.; Kreuter, M.W. Using narrative communication as a tool for health behavior change: A conceptual, theoretical, and empirical overview. *Health Educ. Behav.* **2007**, *34*, 777–792. [CrossRef] [PubMed]
35. BBC News, Coronavirus: Patient Urges People to Be Careful. Available online: https://www.bbc.com/news/av/uk-england-tyne-52028252/coronavirus-patient-urges-people-to-be-careful (accessed on 15 May 2020).

36. The Japan Times, Running Out of Beds and Gear, Tokyo Medical Staff Say Japan's "State of Emergency" Already Here. Available online: https://www.japantimes.co.jp/news/2020/04/07/national/science-health/hospital-beds-gear-coronavirus/#.Xr56WMDgouU (accessed on 15 May 2020).
37. Sibony, A.-L. The UK COVID-19 Response: A Behavioural Irony? *Eur. J. Risk Regul.* **2020**, 1–11. [CrossRef]
38. Moyer-Gusé, E.; Nabi, R.L. Explaining the effects of narrative in an entertainment television program: Overcoming resistance to persuasion. *Hum. Commun. Res.* **2010**, *36*, 26–52. [CrossRef]
39. Gardner, L.; Leshner, G. The Role of Narrative and Other-Referencing in Attenuating Psychological Reactance to Diabetes Self-Care Messages. *Health Commun.* **2016**, *31*, 738–751. [CrossRef] [PubMed]
40. Reynolds-Tylus, T. Psychological Reactance and Persuasive Health Communication: A Review of the Literature. *Front. Commun.* **2019**, *4*, 56. [CrossRef]
41. Griskevicius, V.; Goldstein, N.J.; Mortensen, C.R.; Sundie, J.M.; Cialdini, R.B.; Kenrick, D.T. Fear and loving in las vegas: Evolution, emotion, and persuasion. *J. Mark. Res.* **2009**, *46*, 384–395. [CrossRef]
42. Shah, J.Y. The automatic pursuit and management of goals. *Curr. Dir. Psychol. Sci.* **2005**, *14*, 10–13. [CrossRef]
43. Befu, H. A Critique of the Group Model of Japanese Society. *Soc. Anal.* **1988**, *6*, 29–43.
44. MacFerran, B. Social Norms, Beliefs, and Health. In *Behavioral Economics and Public Health*; Roberto, A., Kawachi, I., Eds.; Oxford University Press: New York, NY, USA, 2015; pp. 133–160.
45. Stok, F.M.; Verkooijen, K.T.; de Ridder, D.T.D.; de Wit, J.B.F.; de Vet, E. How norms work: Self-identification, attitude, and self-efficacy mediate the relation between descriptive social norms and vegetable intake. *Appl. Psychol. Heal. Well-Being* **2014**, *6*, 230–250. [CrossRef]
46. Shen, L. Antecedents to psychological reactance: The impact of threat, message frame, and choice. *Health Commun.* **2015**, *30*, 975–985. [CrossRef]
47. Thrasher, J.F.; Swayampakala, K.; Borland, R.; Nagelhout, G.; Yong, H.H.; Hammond, D.; Bansal-Travers, M.; Thompson, M.; Hardin, J. Influences of Self-Efficacy, Response Efficacy, and Reactance on Responses to Cigarette Health Warnings: A Longitudinal Study of Adult Smokers in Australia and Canada. *Health Commun.* **2016**, *31*, 1517–1526. [CrossRef] [PubMed]
48. Leask, J.; Hooker, C.; King, C. Media coverage of health issues and how to work more effectively with journalists: A qualitative study. *BMC Public Health* **2010**, *10*, 535. [CrossRef] [PubMed]
49. Jones, J.H.; Salathé, M. Early assessment of anxiety and behavioral response to novel swine-origin influenza a(H1N1). *PLoS ONE* **2009**, *4*, e8032. [CrossRef] [PubMed]
50. Iorfa, S.K.; Ottu, I.F.A.; Oguntayo, R.; Ayandele, O.; Kolawole, S.O.; Gandi, J.C.; Dangiwa, A.L.; Olapegba, P.O. COVID-19 knowledge, riskperception and precautionary behaviour among Nigerians: A moderated mediation approach. *MedRxiv* **2020**. [CrossRef]
51. Gustafson, P.E. Gender differences in risk perception: Theoretical and methodological perspectives. *Risk Anal.* **1998**, *18*, 805–811. [CrossRef]
52. Kang, N.E.; Yoon, W.C. Age- and experience-related user behavior differences in the use of complicated electronic devices. *Int. J. Hum. Comput. Stud.* **2008**, *66*, 425–437. [CrossRef]
53. Almutairi, K.M.; Al Helih, E.M.; Moussa, M.; Boshaiqah, A.E.; Saleh Alajilan, A.; Vinluan, J.M.; Almutairi, A. Awareness, Attitudes, and Practices Related to Coronavirus Pandemic among Public in Saudi Arabia. *Fam. Community Health* **2015**, *38*, 332–340. [CrossRef]
54. Cui, B.; Liao, Q.; Lam, W.W.T.; Liu, Z.P.; Fielding, R. Avian influenza A/H7N9 risk perception, information trust and adoption of protective behaviours among poultry farmers in Jiangsu Province, China. *BMC Public Health* **2017**, *17*, 463. [CrossRef]
55. Mccullock, S.P.; Perrault, E.K. Exploring the Effects of Source Credibility and Message Framing on STI Screening Intentions: An Application of Prospect and Protection Motivation Theory. *J. Health Commun.* **2020**, *25*, 1–11. [CrossRef]

Publisher's Note: MDPI stays neutral with regard to jurisdictional claims in published maps and institutional affiliations.

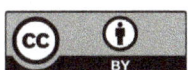

© 2020 by the authors. Licensee MDPI, Basel, Switzerland. This article is an open access article distributed under the terms and conditions of the Creative Commons Attribution (CC BY) license (http://creativecommons.org/licenses/by/4.0/).

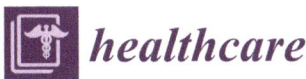

Article

Older Adults' Avoidance of Public Transportation after the Outbreak of COVID-19: Korean Subway Evidence

Byungjin Park [1] and Joonmo Cho [2,*]

[1] HRD Center, Department of Economics, Sungkyunkwan University, Seoul 03063, Korea; park0420jin@g.skku.edu
[2] Department of Economics, Sungkyunkwan University, Seoul 03063, Korea
* Correspondence: trustcho@skku.edu

Abstract: With the spread of the coronavirus worldwide, nations have implemented policies restricting the movement of people to minimize the possibility of infection. Although voluntary restriction is a key factor in reducing mobility, it has only been emphasized in terms of the effect of governments' mobility restriction measures. This research aimed to analyze voluntary mass transportation use after the severe acute respiratory syndrome coronavirus 2 (SARS-CoV-2) outbreak by age group to explore how the perception of the risk of infection affected the public transit system. Mass transportation big data of Seoul Metro transportation use in the capital city of Korea was employed for panel analyses. The analysis results showed that in the period with both the highest and lowest number of infections of SARS-CoV-2, users aged 65 years and over reduced their subway use more than people aged between 20 and 64. This study also found that the decrease in subway use caused by the sharp increase of coronavirus disease 2019 (COVID-19) cases was the most prominent among people aged 65 years and over. The results imply that the elders' avoidance of public transportation affected their daily lives, consumption, and production activities, as well as their mobility.

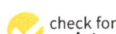

Citation: Park, B.; Cho, J. Older Adults' Avoidance of Public Transportation after the Outbreak of COVID-19: Korean Subway Evidence. *Healthcare* **2021**, *9*, 448. https://doi.org/10.3390/healthcare9040448

Academic Editors: Manoj Sharma and Kavita Batra

Received: 24 February 2021
Accepted: 8 April 2021
Published: 11 April 2021

Publisher's Note: MDPI stays neutral with regard to jurisdictional claims in published maps and institutional affiliations.

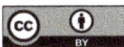

Copyright: © 2021 by the authors. Licensee MDPI, Basel, Switzerland. This article is an open access article distributed under the terms and conditions of the Creative Commons Attribution (CC BY) license (https://creativecommons.org/licenses/by/4.0/).

Keywords: COVID-19; avoidance of infection; social distancing; free tickets for the aged; subway use demand

1. Introduction

Since the World Health Organization (WHO) declared the coronavirus disease 2019 (COVID-19) pandemic, the spread of infections around the world has not abated. While the total number of global COVID-19 cases was 0.7 million in March 2020 when the WHO announced the COVID-19 outbreak a global pandemic, the number of cases exceeded 79.2 million in December 2020 [1,2]. With the incessant outbreaks of community transmission, clusters of cases, and sporadic infections, coronavirus is still spreading throughout the world.

The spread of severe acute respiratory syndrome coronavirus 2 (SARS-CoV-2) infections was inevitable, even in Korea. Figure 1 shows the progress of COVID-19 cases in Seoul, the capital of Korea, between February and September. As of December 24, the number of COVID-19 cases in South Korea reached 53,533, with 756 deaths, and the incidence rate (i.e., the cumulative number of confirmed cases per 100,000 population) was 103.25 [3].

With the spread of the coronavirus worldwide, nations implemented policies restricting the movement of people to minimize the amount of contact between people, as WHO reported that COVID-19 is rapidly transmitted through human contact and respiratory organs [4]. Asymptomatic "silent spreaders" were found, making it difficult to track the routes of transmission [5]. Wuhan, the Chinese city where the pandemic is believed to have started, was effectively sealed off from the rest of the country immediately, and movement between regions in China was strictly banned [6]. In Europe, strict restrictions, such as lockdowns, curfews, and permits for movement, were imposed by governments [7]. In the United States, which has the most coronavirus cases worldwide, heightened mobility restrictions, such as stay-at-home orders, bans on gathering, and travel restrictions, were implemented, depending on the status of each state [8].

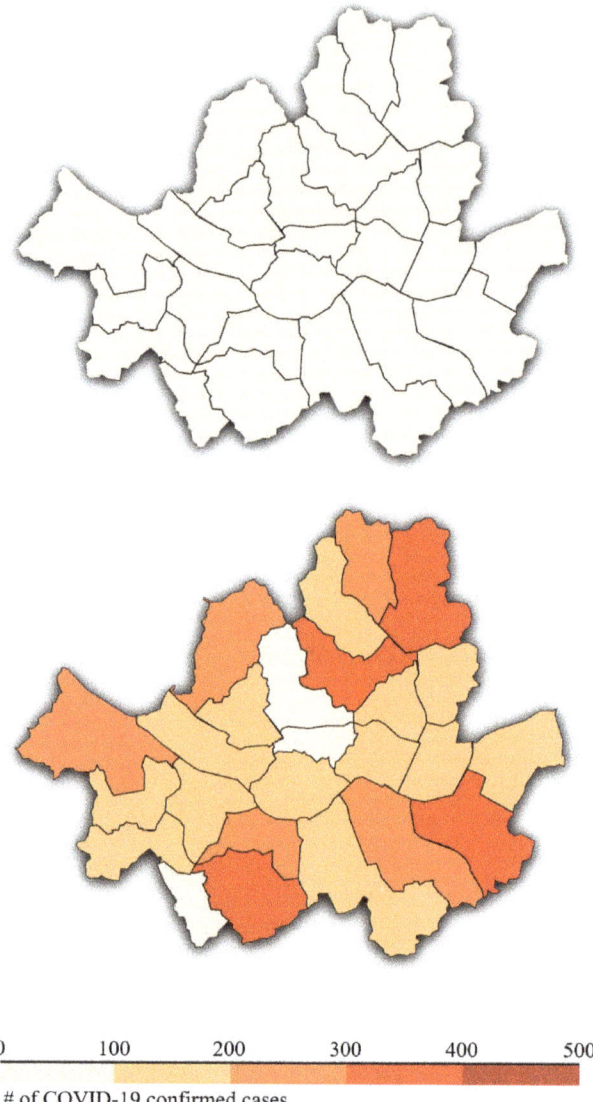

Figure 1. Number of cumulative confirmed cases in Seoul in 2020. The upper and lower figures show the number of infections in February and September, respectively.

The Korean government implemented social distancing measures instead of strong restrictions on movement to curb the contagion of SARS-CoV-2. The call for social distancing is a campaign, guidance, or recommendation of the Korean government to achieve regulated mobility through citizens' voluntary cooperation and compliance. In social distancing phases 1 and 1.5, it was recommended to wear a mask, report meetings and events, and work from home for one-fifth of each institution. In phase 2, all meetings with more than 100 people were prohibited, and a third of employees were encouraged to work from home. Furthermore, the use of entertainment facilities was prohibited and the reduction of store operating hours to 9 p.m. was applied. In phases 2.5 and 3, all of the above restrictions applied to more facilities.

The mobility restriction policies of countries and voluntary restrictions, which were driven by the fear of the coronavirus infection, have led to a decrease in transit demand. In France, consumer mobility, which was estimated based on the use of payment cards, decreased by 75% during the national lockdown compared to 2019 [9]. According to Google Trend data, mass transit demand in ten countries, including Italy, Brazil, and the United Kingdom, fell sharply since the COVID-19 outbreak [10]. In Mexico, the use of automobiles decreased by 10 to 25% since the outbreak [11].

Seoul has also witnessed a drastic reduction of transit demand amid the pandemic, which can be measured based on the changes in mass transit system use in Seoul, which is among the top ten in the world in terms of efficiency and user satisfaction [12]. The population of Seoul was 9,668,465 as of December 2020, and the number of uses of buses and subways surpassed 100 million each month. Figure 2 shows the number of bus and subway rides in 2018, 2019, and 2020. As the number of cases of COVID-19 began to rise in late January 2020, mass transit demand fell dramatically and rebounded after March, but it was still well below the demand recorded in the same periods of 2018 and 2019. Furthermore, in August, the mass transportation demand declined again after the outbreak of cluster infections in Seoul, showing that mass transportation was significantly affected by the pandemic. Statistics on bus and subway use are in Table A1 of the Appendix A.

Most studies on the decrease of mass transit demand are focused on the effect of governments' mobility restriction measures. However, there is a lack of studies on the impact of the voluntary restriction that significantly affected the decrease in transit demand. This may be attributed to the fact that, as many countries are implementing restrictions on mobility, it is difficult to isolate the effect of citizens' voluntary restraint of movement.

Data on subway transit demand in Seoul is useful for studying the voluntary mobility reduction during the pandemic since it has three characteristics that are not found in other cities. First, it is a type of mass transit that carries a high probability of infection. Mass transportation involves very high risks of infection because of the high density, diversity of contacts, and potential presence of patients [13]. Hence, when traveling in the subway, passengers are aware of the risk of infection. Second, the government did not issue any specific restrictions on subway use. Without enforced mobility regulation, subway use reflects the voluntary mobility of people. Third, people aged 65 and over in Seoul can ride a subway for free due to Article 19 of the Welfare of Senior Citizens Act [14]. For the elderly without income earned through economic activity participation, the subway is an essential and the most common means of mass transit for leisure.

However, after the COVID-19 outbreak, subways were classified as facilities that carried the highest infection risk, and the age group most prone to fatality because of a SARS-CoV-2 infection is the elderly group. Therefore, though they have free access to the subway, i.e., the most efficient means of movement, the aged cannot ride on a subway train without concern regarding COVID-19's impact. As such, the change in the subway ride patterns by the elderly most effectively reflects the perception of the risk of the COVID-19 infection.

The pandemic negatively affected the labor market, as well as people's perceptions of the risk of infection. At the outbreak of Middle East Respiratory Syndrome, the older adults were the most vulnerable in the labor market, and the confusion in the urban labor market was greater than in the rural areas [15,16]. With the prolonged period of the COVID-19 pandemic, the deterioration of the labor market caused a decline in people's consumption and income. These changes eventually lead to mobility changes.

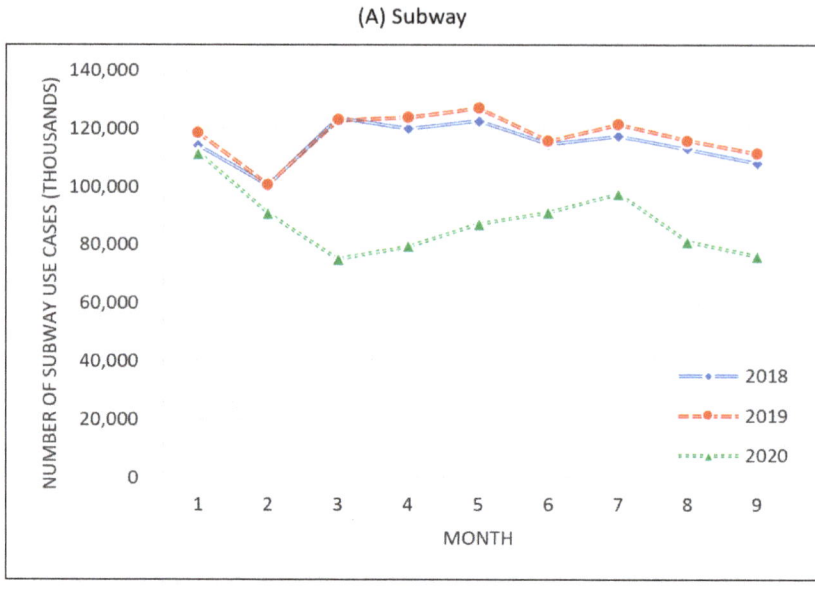

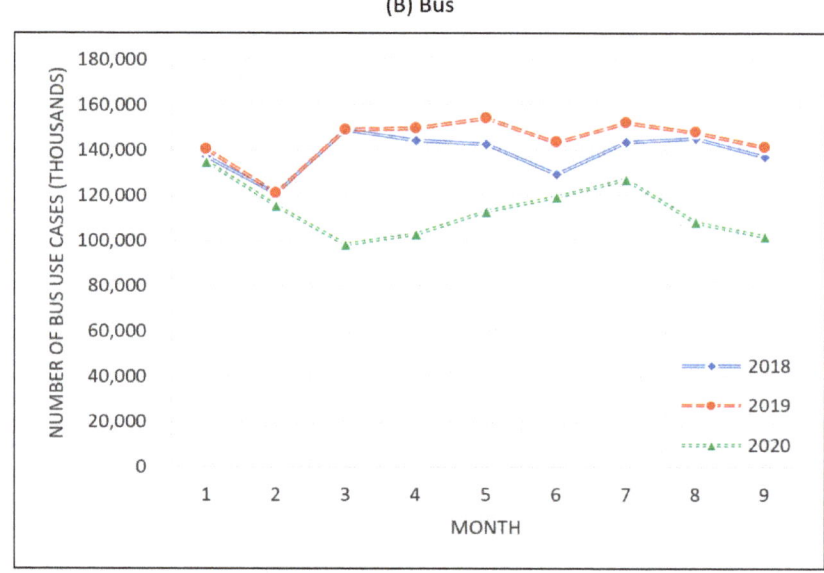

Figure 2. Number of uses of mass transit during 2018–2020.

This study aimed to empirically analyze the changes in subway use patterns by the elderly and the economically active population amid the risk of SARS-CoV-2 infection. First, the period when cases spiked sharply was separated from other periods for the analysis. The Korean government controlled the social distancing level according to the number of cases. The rise of the social distancing level imposed by the government was intended to heighten citizens' awareness of the pandemic and cause behavioral change. As such, by focusing on the social distancing level imposed in each period, changes in the behavior of each age group associated with the changes in the social distancing level can be identified. Next, the elasticity of the demand for subway use in response to the number of COVID-19 cases was measured to determine whether the elderly, who are most vulnerable to the coronavirus, were more sensitive to the risk of infection than young people. Lastly, through analysis based on the number of subway stations by period, this study attempted to determine whether changes in subway ride decisions were related to the fear of SARS-CoV-2 infection. In areas near transfer stations (the number of transfer stations was counted based on the number of subway lines available for the station; for instance, for a subway station on three subway lines, the number of stations was counted as three) and multiple stations, there was more transit demand because of easy access to the subway. That is, such areas carry a higher risk of infection from more human contacts. Accordingly, if areas with a greater number of stations are found to experience a higher decrease in passengers than areas with a smaller number of stations, that can be interpreted as a behavioral change to avoid SARS-CoV-2 infection.

Change in the Pattern of Subway Use Demand Amid the Pandemic in Seoul

The number of deaths because of SARS-CoV-2 infection rises as the age of patients climbs. According to the Center for Disease Control and Prevention data, 80% of deaths from the coronavirus are associated with people over 65 years old [17]. Reports on the case fatality rate (CFR) in China and Italy found that the CFR for people aged under 60 was less than 2%, while the CFR for the aged over 60 years old was 20% [18]. In the United States, the CFR of those aged 65 or older was 3 to 27%, higher than that of younger people [19]. In Korea, the COVID-19-related CFR for the elderly was like other countries. Figure 3 shows the share of Korean coronavirus cases and CFR by age group. Over 70% of people infected with COVID-19 were aged under 50, whereas the CFR showed a rapid nonlinear rise for people aged over 60. Figure 4 shows the incidence rate of the coronavirus by age group. The number of confirmed cases per 100,000 population was relatively high among the elderly aged 60 or older.

The COVID-19 pandemic has led to changes in the hours of subway use and the number of rides. Figure 5 shows a change in the share of the number of subway rides by the hour in 2020 and 2019. Compared with 2019, the number of subway rides of passengers aged 20 to 64 in 2020 rose by 0.2% to 1% during 6–9 a.m. (commute to work) and rose by 0.5 to 0.9% during 5–6 p.m. (commute from work). In hours other than those, the use of the subway transit dropped. This was likely to be attributed to the reduction of operating hours of stores owing to the social distancing rule and a decrease in the number of permitted persons for meetings and dinners. The subway use for passengers aged 65 and over rose by 0.5% during 5–7 a.m., and the use of the subway decreased during hours other than this. Such changes in time for the use of the subway for the aged people who were not constrained by time for their social activities seemed to be meant to reduce human contact and restrict external activities voluntarily to avoid SARS-CoV-2 infection.

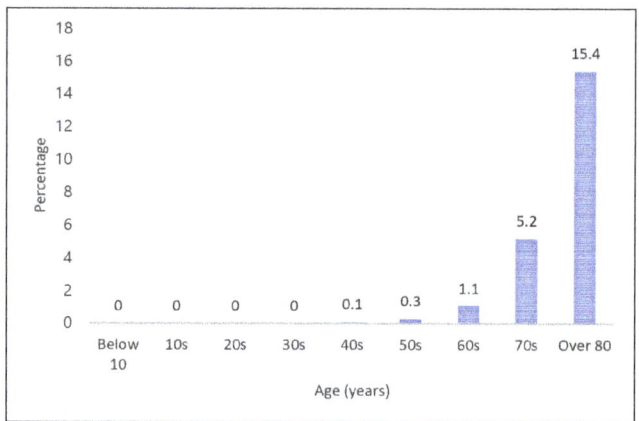

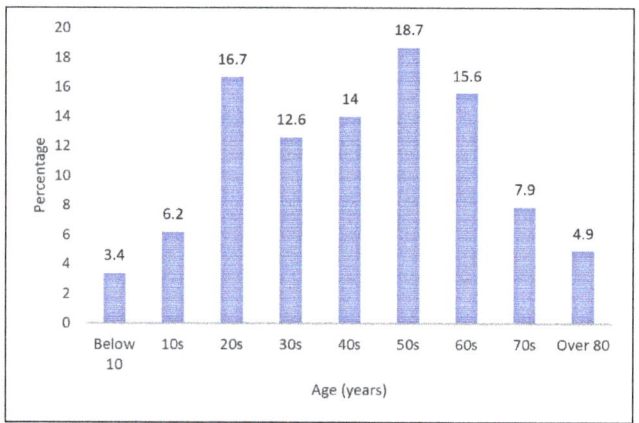

Figure 3. COVID-19 status in South Korea as of 24 December 2020.

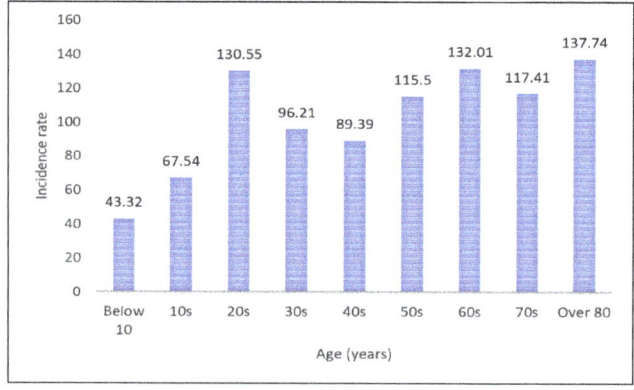

Figure 4. Incidence rate per 100,000 in South Korea as of 24 December 2020.

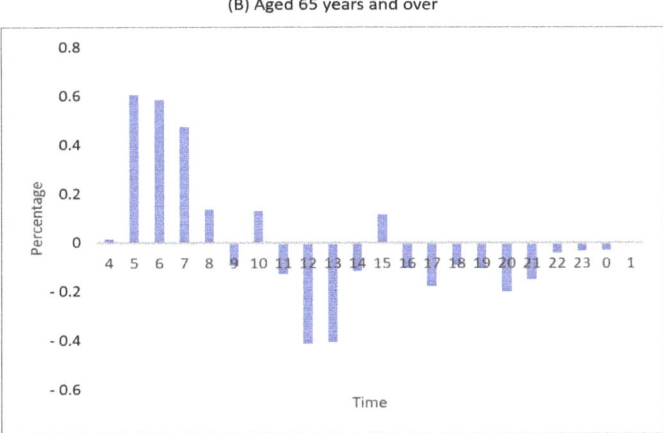

Figure 5. Change in the share of subway use hours.

2. Materials and Methods

2.1. Data

This study collected data from the Seoul Bigdata Campus and the Seoul Open Data Plaza of the Seoul Metropolitan government. The period for this analysis ran from January to September in 2018, 2019, and 2020. Data for the cases of COVID-19 in Seoul relied on data from the Seoul Metropolitan government and the data for the Korean cases were from the Center for Systems Science and Engineering of Johns Hopkins University.

2.1.1. Seoul Bigdata Campus

The Seoul Bigdata Campus collects big data provided by organizations of the Seoul Metropolitan government and provides it to public institutions, academics, and private companies to help with research and solve social issues. As the collected data contains personal information, the sources of that data needed to be visited to get the preprocessing and approval for exporting that data before it can be used. Figure 6 shows the procedure of using raw data obtained from the Seoul Bigdata Campus.

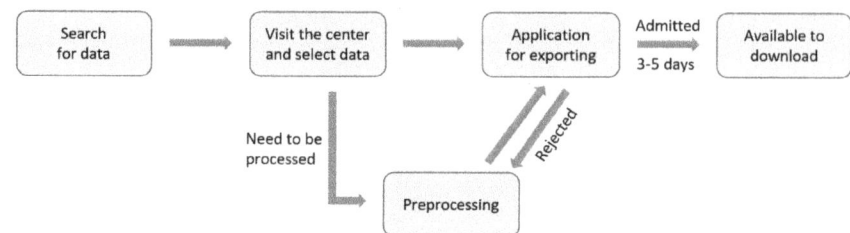

Figure 6. Data collection procedure of the Seoul Bigdata Campus.

The data on subway use in Seoul was the raw data provided by Tmoney Co., Ltd. to the Seoul Bigdata Campus, which could not be used without preprocessing and approval for exporting it. In Seoul, passengers must use smart cards equipped with a transportation card function to use the subway, and thus data from Tmoney Co., Ltd. that lists the details of the transportation card transactions are highly reliable. This data includes the date and time for the subway use, the station for departure and arrival, the type of subway user (type of subway user refers to senior citizens, persons of national merit, children, foreign senior citizens, general citizens, disabled persons, and youth; about 80% of subway users are general citizens aged between 20 and 64, the elderly aged 65 and older account for 12 to 13% of users, and the rest account for 6 to 7%), and the number of passengers.

This research focused on the changes in demand for the subway from residents in Seoul. While Seoul Metro also covers subway stations in both Seoul Metropolitan City and Gyeonggi-do province, this study conducted analysis only for subway stations located in 25 districts of Seoul Metropolitan City and collected data of the Korea Smart Card Co. on the number of rides by the district at departure stations.

2.1.2. Seoul Open Data Plaza

Like the Seoul Bigdata Campus, Seoul Open Data Plaza collects data provided by organizations of the Seoul Metropolitan government. However, unlike Seoul Bigdata Campus, it makes public data open to all citizens and does not require visits to organizations providing such data. Seoul Open Data Plaza provides links to providers of a vast amount of data such that the latest data can be obtained from the links. Data for independent variables used in this study were based on the data of Seoul Open Data Plaza, the Ministry of Land, Infrastructure, and Transport, and the Transport Operation and Information Service of Seoul.

2.2. Empirical Model

This study used panel data of 25 districts in Seoul. Analyses were conducted in Stata/SE (version 16.1, StataCorp., College Station, TX, USA). Using the fixed-effects model, changes in the pattern of subway use by passengers aged 20 to 64 and passengers aged 65 and older amid the COVID-19 pandemic were analyzed. Fixed-effects models are effective at controlling for omitted variable bias because of unobserved heterogeneity [20]. Hence, this kind of model was suitable for controlling the environmental characteristics of each district of Seoul Metropolitan City.

The Korean government adjusted the social distancing levels based on variations of the number of confirmed cases. In phase 2 or higher of social distancing, there were significantly more restrictions on the economically active population than below phase 2. Hence, it was necessary to distinguish the period according to the social distancing level. The formula was as follows:

$$y_{it} = \beta_1 \text{SDLv1} + \beta_2 \text{SDLv2} + \beta_3 \text{CarSpeed}_{it} + \beta_4 \text{Pop}_{it} + \beta_5 \text{OwnCar}_{it} + \beta_6 \text{Wealth}_{it} + \alpha_i + \varepsilon_{it}. \quad (1)$$

In Formula (1) above, subscript i means the districts of Seoul and t refers to the monthly data. y_{it} is the logarithm of the number of subway rides per month in each district. SDLv1 is a dummy variable taking 1 for January, February, May, June, and July 2020 when social distancing was in phase 1 to 1.5 and taking 0 for other periods. SDLv2 is a dummy variable taking 1 for March, April, August, and September of 2020 when social distancing was at phase 2 or higher and taking 0 for other periods. CarSpeed is the average speed of automobiles measured by each district. Pop refers to the population registered in each district office. OwnCar refers to the share of privately owned cars out of the total registered vehicles in each district. Wealth is the average price per square meter of an apartment house in each district. α_i refers to the time-invariant location fixed effects. β_i and ε_{it} are coefficients and error term respectively.

Next, the elasticity of subway use in response to the number of COVID-19 cases was measured. The elasticity indicates the sensitivity of the number of subway uses in response to an increase in cases, and also reveals the differing sensitivity to the number of cases among age groups. The formula was as follows:

$$y_{it} = \beta_1 \text{Covid}_t + \beta_2 \text{CarSpeed}_{it} + \beta_3 \text{Pop}_{it} + \beta_4 \text{OwnCar}_{it} + \beta_5 \text{Wealth}_{it} + \alpha_i + \varepsilon_{it}. \quad (2)$$

Additionally, concerning the Covid variable, the number of cases in Seoul and the number of cases in Korea were used to see the differences between residents' responses to infection in local communities and nationwide, respectively.

Last, if the decrease in mass transit demand was due to the perception of the risk of the infection from the coronavirus, regions with a higher subway demand would experience a larger decrease in subway use. Areas with a large number of subway stations and transfer stations have a higher demand for subway use than other areas due to better accessibility to subways. The high demand for subway use not only increases the population density but also increases the floating population. This environment makes it easier for people to be more exposed to SARS-CoV-2 infection. Accordingly, analysis by period was made separately for areas with 16 or more stations, including transfer stations, and areas with less than 16 stations.

3. Results

The Seoul Metropolitan Subway with a potentially higher rate of SARS-CoV-2 cluster infections saw the number of users declining significantly since the outbreak of the pandemic. Figure 7 shows the changes in the number of rides for passengers aged between 20 and 64 and those aged 65 and older. During 2018 and 2019 before the pandemic, those aged between 20 and 64 took 94,130,730 subway rides a month on average, and those aged 65 and older took 14,278,200 rides per month. After the COVID-19 outbreak, people between 20 and 64 used the subway 72,398,975 times a month while those aged 65 and older used the subway 10,815,514 times a month, showing a dramatic decrease.

Table 1 shows the change in the number of subway rides in each age group. Under stronger social distancing levels, the subway use of the two groups decreased. People aged 20 to 64 decreased their number of subway rides by 13% in phases 1 and 1.5 of social distancing, and by 30% as the social distancing level rose to phase 2 or higher. Likewise, the elderly aged 65 and older reduced their subway use by 19% in phases 1 and 1.5 and by 42% in phase 2 or higher. This suggests changes in the users' behavioral patterns to avoid cluster infection risk by reducing subway use during the periods when the number of cases of the coronavirus increased, and thus the social distancing level was heightened.

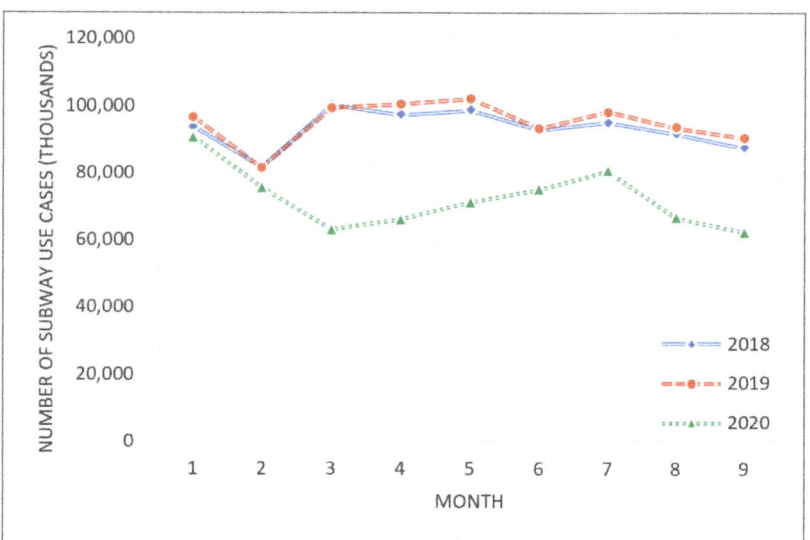

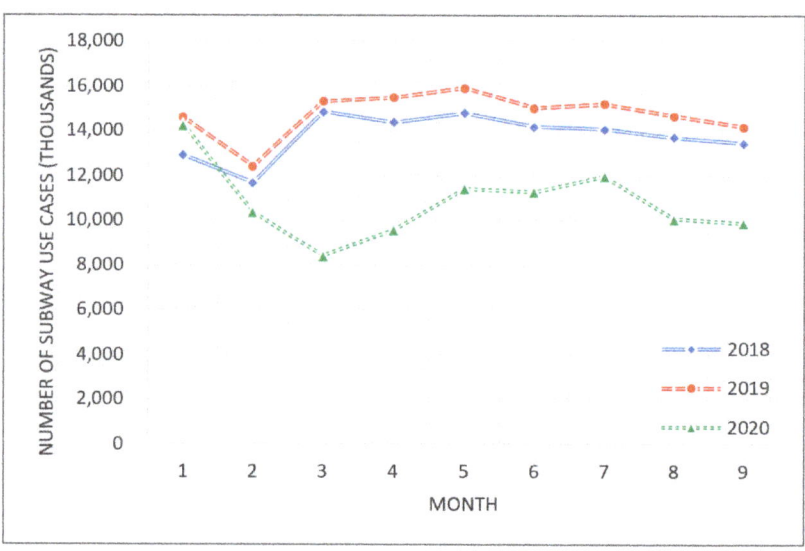

Figure 7. Number of subway uses during 2018–2020.

Table 1. Panel results: change in the subway demand by age and period.

Independent Variable	Dependent Variable	
	Log(Number of Subway Use Cases)	
	Aged 20 to 64 Years Old	Over 65 Years Old
Social distancing level 1 period	−0.1301 *** (0.0143)	−0.1973 *** (0.0109)
Social distancing level 2 period	−0.3092 *** (0.0208)	−0.4212 *** (0.0158)
Average car speed	−0.0309 *** (0.0061)	−0.0437 *** (0.0045)
Population	0.0016 (0.0011)	−0.0009 (0.0013)
Percentage of cars that were privately owned	−0.0314 ** (0.0146)	−0.0006 (0.0079)
Average apartment price per square meter	−0.0001 * (0.0000)	0.0002 *** (0.0000)
Cons	18.0675 *** (1.3860)	14.3751 *** (0.7550)
R-squared	0.7674	0.7782
Observations	675	675
Location Fixed Effect	Yes	Yes

Note: Cluster robust standard errors are given in parenthesis. * $p < 0.1$, ** $p < 0.05$, *** $p < 0.01$.

Although the subway use demand decreased in both the 20–64 years and 65+ years age groups, the subway use of the elderly fell more prominently regardless of the social distancing phase. For the economically active population of Seoul, the subway is an essential transportation means to commute to work. Accordingly, this study expected that in phase 1 of social distancing, the decrease in subway use demand by people aged 20 to 64 years would be smaller than that for the elderly aged 65 years and older, and this expectation was consistent with analysis results. When the social distancing level was lifted to phase 2 or higher, the subway use demand by the economically active population decreased by a larger margin than for people aged 65 years and older due to activity-related reasons, such as remote work and a ban on nonessential meetings and events. Nevertheless, in phase 2 or higher of social distancing, subway use demand by people aged 65 years and older dropped by a significantly larger margin than the economically active population. For the elderly, the strengthening of social distancing did not change much in daily life, but the increase in the possibility of SARS-CoV-2 infection caused decision-making changes. Therefore, the result implies that the subway use demand by people aged 65 years and older was affected more by the voluntary restraint of mobility to avoid coronavirus infection than the social distancing policy.

Table 2 shows the change in subway use in tandem with the increase in the number of coronavirus cases. Both in Seoul and Korea as a whole, the increase in the number of coronavirus cases was negatively related to subway use. However, subway use was more sensitive to the number of cases in Seoul than to the number of cases nationwide. For subway users aged 20 to 64 years, a 1% increase in the number of Seoul cases led to a decrease in subway use by 0.06%, but a 1% increase in the number of cases nationwide reduced subway use by 0.03%. As for the elderly aged 65 years and older, the elasticity of subway use was higher in response to the number of cases in both Seoul and the whole nation than for people aged 20 to 64 years. A 1% increase in the number of Seoul cases reduced subway use by 0.08%, while a 1% increase in the number cases nationwide led to a decrease in subway rides by 0.06%. This finding suggests that despite the differing elasticities of subway use in response to the number of cases in a given region and the nation as a whole, the sensitivity to the risk of SARS-CoV-2 infection was higher for the aged people than for the younger people.

Table 2. Panel results: elasticity of subway use demand by age in response to the number of COVID-19 cases.

Independent Variable	Dependent Variable			
	Log (the Number of Subway Use Cases)			
	Aged 20 to 64 Years Old		Over 65 Years Old	
Log(number of cases in Seoul)	−0.0600 *** (0.0051)	-	−0.0810 *** (0.0048)	-
Log(number of cases in Korea)	-	−0.0357 *** (0.0022)	-	−0.0627 *** (0.0022)
Average car speed	−0.0252 *** (0.0044)	−0.0315 *** (0.0046)	−0.0501 *** (0.0034)	−0.0410 *** (0.0029)
Population	−0.0002 (0.0029)	0.0016 (0.0020)	−0.0057 * (0.0033)	−0.0028 (0.0020)
Percentage of cars that were privately owned	0.0284 (0.0344)	−0.0323 (0.0430)	0.1656 *** (0.0395)	0.0871 ** (0.0410)
Average apartment price per squre meter	0.0001 (0.0001)	−0.0008 *** (0.0001)	0.0008 *** (0.0002)	−0.0000 (0.0001)
Cons	12.8778 *** (3.1716)	18.9296 *** (3.7799)	0.4762 (3.4244)	7.2712 * (3.5412)
R-squared	0.5893	0.6058	0.5671	0.7323
Observations	225	225	225	225
Location Fixed Effect	Yes	Yes	Yes	Yes

Note: Cluster robust standard errors are given in parenthesis. * $p < 0.1$, ** $p < 0.05$, *** $p < 0.01$.

The results of the analysis given above confirmed that subway use demand decreased because of the coronavirus and that the aged were more sensitive to the risks associated with the virus than other age groups. Table 3 illustrates the analysis results by area based on the number of subway stations, including transfer stations. The findings revealed that the change in subway use pattern to avoid the infection risk was similar in all areas. Passengers aged 65 years and older decreased their number of subway rides more than those aged 20 to 64 years, regardless of the number of subway stations. Moreover, the elderly reduced their number of subway rides by a larger margin in areas with 16 or more stations, including transfer stations, than in areas with less than 16 stations. Both groups showed a greater drop in mass transit demand in areas with a large number of subway stations. This implies that people were trying to avoid high-risk areas.

Table 3. Panel results: change in the subway use demand with respect to the number of subway stations.

Independent Variable	Dependent Variable			
	Log (Number of Subway Use Cases)			
	Less than 16 Stations		At Least 16 Stations	
	Aged 20–64	Over 65	Aged 20–64	Over 65
Social distancing level 1	−0.1211 *** (0.0185)	−0.1751 *** (0.0109)	−0.1462 *** (0.0155)	−0.2193 *** (0.0146)
Social distancing level 2	−0.2928 *** (0.0301)	−0.3877 *** (0.0164)	−0.3349 *** (0.0227)	−0.4538 *** (0.0197)
Average car speed	−0.0287 *** (0.0069)	−0.0500 *** (0.0081)	−0.0304 *** (0.0085)	−0.0386 *** (0.0059)
Population	0.0009 (0.0015)	−0.0017 ** (0.0007)	0.0016 (0.0020)	−0.0006 (0.0032)
Percentage of cars that were privately owned	0.0335 (0.0358)	−0.0072 (0.0223)	−0.0462 *** (0.0131)	−0.0021 (0.0112)
Average apartment price per squre meter	−0.0002 ** (0.0000)	0.0001 ** (0.0000)	−0.0000 (0.0000)	0.0002 *** (0.0000)
Cons	11.9597 *** (3.0686)	15.2013 *** (2.0075)	19.7357 *** (1.3862)	14.4994 *** (1.1523)
R-squared	0.7617	0.7740	0.7833	0.7861
Observations	351	351	324	324
Location Fixed Effect	Yes	Yes	Yes	Yes

Note: Cluster robust standard errors are given in parenthesis. ** $p < 0.05$, *** $p < 0.01$.

4. Discussion

The results of this study showed the change in subway use demand in Seoul after the outbreak of SARS-CoV-2. The significant decrease in mass transit demand in both groups suggested that people's mobility was greatly affected by the risk of infection. In particular, people aged 65 years and over avoided using the subway more than those aged between 20 and 64 years. The sensitivity to the risk of SARS-CoV-2 infection was also found to be high in the elderly. This suggests that because of the high fatality rate from the coronavirus among the elderly, the elderly's fear of the pandemic was stronger, leading to an avoidance of public transportation. In sum, this study suggests that the differences in perceptions of the risk of coronavirus varied with age, and this was manifested through their mobility changes. The decline in people's mobility cannot be interpreted as just an evasive behavior due to the risk of coronavirus infection. The decrease in spaces of consumption can be one factor that reduces mobility. These include a meeting cancellation, store closures, prohibition of leisure activities, and so on. The deteriorating labor market conditions can also contribute to the change of mobility. A decrease in income due to unemployment would shrink the amount of consumption, which can lead to a decline in mobility. There can be many other factors that can cause changes in human mobility. In this study, we focused on the overall change in people's mobility by age. Therefore, if the socioeconomic factors mentioned above can be analyzed with mobility changes, we believe that the effect of infection risk on mobility reduction can be identified in detail. Furthermore, through an analysis of the relationship between mobility and the regional economic damage due to the coronavirus, we will be able to find the link between the consumption pattern and human mobility.

5. Conclusions

As the COVID-19 pandemic is protracted for an extended period, cases of COVID-19 are found in all age groups, but a high case fatality rate is still concentrated in the elderly.

This means that in older adults, a coronavirus infection is more likely to result in the loss of life. In this respect, the difference in the human mobility between the young and the elderly presented in this study can be said to be a natural result. However, human mobility is associated with socioeconomic activities; therefore, it is difficult to explain the change in mobility solely in terms of the coronavirus risk. In order to analyze the effects of the coronavirus in more detail, an analysis of factors by age will be needed.

The Korean government is implementing a subsidy policy and plans to give additional subsidies to help small business owners who are suffering due to the COVID-19 pandemic. Since not all small business owners have suffered the same damage, the controversy over the target of the COVID-19 subsidy is increasing. The biggest impact for small business owners is the decline in sales due to people's reduced mobility. Mobility encompasses various types of movement for living, leisure, consumption, and production. Therefore, if there is a regional analysis using the big data based on the result of mobility changes of this study, it will be helpful for the government to decide upon a subsidy policy.

Author Contributions: B.P. contributed to the data collection, statistical analyses, and the literature search strategy. J.C. contributed to the conceptual framework and writing the paper. Both authors contributed to the interpretation of the data, revised the article, and approved the published version of the manuscript. All authors have read and agreed to the published version of the manuscript.

Funding: This paper was supported by SKKU Excellence in Research Award Research Fund, Sungkyunkwan University, 2020.

Institutional Review Board Statement: Not applicable.

Informed Consent Statement: Not applicable.

Data Availability Statement: The data presented in this study are available on request from the corresponding author. The data are not publicly available due to the institutional data policy.

Conflicts of Interest: The authors declare no conflict of interest.

Appendix A

Table A1. Statistics on mass transit use in Seoul during 2018 to 2020.

Age Group	Year	Mean	Min	Max	SD
Subway Use (Number of Rides)					
Total	2018	114,920,221	100,453,195	123,690,832	6,874,797
	2019	117,422,892	100,588,781	126,864,286	7,447,456
	2020	87,755,394	75,018,658	111,563,274	11,061,701
20 to 64 years	2018	93,219,289	81,810,105	100,149,309	5,413,155
	2019	95,042,169	81,525,891	102,024,162	5,930,896
	2020	72,398,975	62,409,113	90,678,007	8,662,742
Over 65 years	2018	13,789,837	11,678,379	14,856,445	944,777
	2019	14,766,562	12,435,456	15,931,192	960,168
	2020	10,815,514	8,410,424	14,265,611	1,587,980
Bus Use (Number of Rides)					
Total	2018	138,688,913	120,557,605	149,004,732	8,411,540
	2019	144,219,373	120,915,659	154,087,859	9,389,018
	2020	113,406,948	98,244,352	134,661,069	11,473,515

References

1. World Health Organization. Coronavirus Disease 2019 (COVID-19) Situation Report—71. 2020. Available online: https://www.who.int/docs/default-source/coronaviruse/situation-reports/20200331-sitrep-71-covid-19.pdf?sfvrsn=4360e92b_8 (accessed on 2 January 2021).
2. World Health Organization. Weekly Epidemiological Update—29 December 2020. 2020. Available online: https://www.who.int/publications/m/item/weekly-epidemiological-update---29-december-2020 (accessed on 2 January 2021).
3. Korea Disease Control and Prevention Agency. Updates on COVID-19 in Republic of Korea (as of 24 December). 2020. Available online: http://ncov.mohw.go.kr/upload/viewer/skin/doc.html?fn=1609113399177_20201228085639.pdf&rs=/upload/viewer/result/202102/ (accessed on 2 January 2021).
4. World Health Organization. Coronavirus Disease (COVID-19): How Is It Transmitted? 2020. Available online: https://www.who.int/emergencies/diseases/novel-coronavirus-2019/question-and-answers-hub/q-a-detail/coronavirus-disease-covid-19-how-is-it-transmitted (accessed on 24 December 2020).
5. Shukman, B.D. Coronavirus: The Mystery of Asymptomatic "Silent Spreaders". BBC News. 2020. Available online: https://www.bbc.com/news/uk-52840763 (accessed on 24 December 2020).
6. Liu, W.; Yue, X.-G.; Tchounwou, P.B. Response to the covid-19 epidemic: The chinese experience and implications for other countries. *Int. J. Environ. Res. Public Health* **2020**, *17*, 2304. [CrossRef] [PubMed]
7. BBC News. Covid: How are European Countries Tackling the Pandemic? 2021. Available online: https://www.bbc.com/news/explainers-53640249 (accessed on 5 February 2021).
8. Bergquist, S.; Otten, T.; Sarich, N. COVID-19 pandemic in the United States. *Health Policy Technol.* **2020**, *9*, 623–638. [CrossRef] [PubMed]
9. Bounie, D.; Camara, Y.; Galbraith, J.W. Consumers' mobility, expenditure and online-offline substitution response to COVID-19: Evidence from French transaction data. *Ssrn Electron. J.* **2020**. [CrossRef]
10. Tirachini, A.; Cats, O. COVID-19 and Public transportation: Current assessment, prospects, and research needs. *J. Public Transp.* **2020**, *22*, 1. [CrossRef]
11. Campos-Vazquez, R.M.; Esquivel, G. Consumption and geographic mobility in pandemic times. Evidence from Mexico. *Rev. Econ. Househ.* **2021**, 1–19. [CrossRef]
12. Knupfer, S.M.; Pokotilo, V.; Woetzel, J. Elements of Success: Urban Transportation Systems of 24 Global Cities. McKinsey&Company, 2018. Available online: https://www.mckinsey.com/~{}/media/McKinsey/Business%20Functions/Sustainability/Our%20Insights/Elements%20of%20success%20Urban%20transportation%20systems%20of%2024%20global%20cities/Urban-transportation-systems_e-versions.ashx (accessed on 2 January 2021).
13. Union Internationale des Transports Publics. Management of COVID-19 Guidelines for Public Transport Operators. 2020. Available online: https://cms.uitp.org/wp/wp-content/uploads/2020/06/Corona-Virus_EN.pdf (accessed on 2 January 2021).
14. Korea Law Information Center. Welfare of Older Persons Act. 2015. Available online: https://www.law.go.kr/LSW/lsInfoP.do?lsiSeq=166670#0000 (accessed on 24 December 2020).
15. Lee, A.; Cho, J. The impact of epidemics on labor market: Identifying victims of the Middle East Respiratory Syndrome in the Korean labor market. *Int. J. Equity Health* **2016**, *15*, 196. [CrossRef] [PubMed]
16. Lee, A.; Cho, J. The impact of city epidemics on rural labor market: The Korean Middle East Respiratory Syndrome case. *Jpn. World Econ.* **2017**, *43*, 30–40. [CrossRef] [PubMed]
17. Centers for Disease Control and Prevention. Older Adults at Greater Risk of Requiring Hospitalization or Dying If Diagnosed with COVID-19. 2020. Available online: https://www.cdc.gov/coronavirus/2019-ncov/need-extra-precautions/older-adults.html (accessed on 20 January 2021).
18. Onder, G.; Rezza, G.; Brusaferro, S. Case-fatality rate and characteristics of patients dying in relation to COVID-19 in Italy. *JAMA* **2020**, *323*, 1775–1776. [CrossRef] [PubMed]
19. Famularo, G. Comment on: COVID-19 and Older Adults: What We Know. *J. Am. Geriatr. Soc.* **2020**, *68*, 2197. [CrossRef] [PubMed]
20. Wooldridge, J.M. *Econometric Analysis of Cross Section and Panel Data*, 2nd ed.; The MIT Press: Cambridge, MA, USA, 2010.

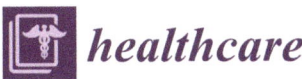

Article

Testing the Multi-Theory Model (MTM) to Predict the Use of New Technology for Social Connectedness in the COVID-19 Pandemic

Manoj Sharma [1], Kavita Batra [2,*] and Jason Flatt [1]

[1] Department of Environmental and Occupational Health, University of Nevada, Las Vegas, NV 89119, USA; Manoj.Sharma@unlv.edu (M.S.); Jason.flatt@unlv.edu (J.F.)
[2] Office of Research, Kirk Kerkorian School of Medicine, University of Nevada, Las Vegas, NV 89102, USA
* Correspondence: Kavita.batra@unlv.edu

Abstract: Loneliness or social isolation, recently described as a "behavioral epidemic," remains a long-standing public health issue, which has worsened during the COVID-19 pandemic. The use of technology has been suggested to enhance social connectedness and to decrease the negative health outcomes associated with social isolation. However, till today, no theory-based studies were performed to examine the determinants of technology use. Therefore, the current study aims to test theory-based determinants in explaining the adoption of new technology in a nationally representative sample during the COVID-19 pandemic (n = 382). A psychometrically reliable and valid instrument based on the multi-theory model (MTM) of health behavior change was administered electronically using a cross-sectional study design. A total of 47.1% of the respondents reported high levels of social isolation, and 40.6% did not use any new technology. Among technology users (59.4%), the three initiation constructs participatory dialogue (b = 0.054, $p < 0.05$), behavioral confidence (b = 0.184, $p < 0.001$), and changes in the physical environment (b= 0.053, $p < 0.05$) were significant and accounted for 38.3% of the variance in the initiation of new technologies. Concerning sustenance in technology users, all three constructs emotional transformation (b = 0.115, $p < 0.001$), practice for change (b = 0.086, $p < 0.001$), and changes in the social environment (b = 0.061, $p < 0.001$) were significant and accounted for 42.6% of the variance in maintaining the use of new technology. MTM offers a powerful framework to design health promotion interventions encouraging the use of new technologies to foster greater social connectedness amid the COVID-19 pandemic and beyond it.

Keywords: social isolation; social connectedness; loneliness; depression; technology; internet; smartphones; m-health; COVID-19; pandemic

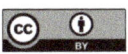

Citation: Sharma, M.; Batra, K.; Flatt, J. Testing the Multi-Theory Model (MTM) to Predict the Use of New Technology for Social Connectedness in the COVID-19 Pandemic. *Healthcare* **2021**, *9*, 838. https://doi.org/10.3390/healthcare9070838

Academic Editor: Francesco Faita

Received: 6 June 2021
Accepted: 28 June 2021
Published: 1 July 2021

Publisher's Note: MDPI stays neutral with regard to jurisdictional claims in published maps and institutional affiliations.

Copyright: © 2021 by the authors. Licensee MDPI, Basel, Switzerland. This article is an open access article distributed under the terms and conditions of the Creative Commons Attribution (CC BY) license (https://creativecommons.org/licenses/by/4.0/).

1. Introduction

Loneliness or perceived social isolation were recently described as a "behavioral epidemic," which has worsened in the wake of the COVID-19 pandemic [1–3]. Loneliness reflects subjective experiences, while social isolation describes the objective state of an individual's social interactions [4,5]. Research has shown that loneliness and social isolation have adverse physical and mental health outcomes. Loneliness and social isolation are associated with an increased risk of depression, cognitive decline, heart disease, stroke, and premature mortality [6–8]. A meta-analysis found that both subjective and objective loneliness or social isolation increases the risk of mortality, with a 26% increased likelihood of mortality for individuals reporting loneliness, 29% for those reporting social isolation, and 32% for those living alone [7]. Moreover, the risk of mortality following loneliness/social isolation was equivalent to the mortality risk among individuals with extreme or severe obesity.

The COVID-19 pandemic has heightened both the public's and public health practitioners' concerns about loneliness and social isolation. Specifically, stay-at-home orders and social distancing measures to reduce the spread of COVID-19 have resulted in people avoiding public spaces and crowds, canceling social activities, and avoiding close contact with others. These preventive behaviors are essential for those at a greater risk of severe illness from COVID-19 and related hospitalization and mortality [9]. Individuals at higher risk for severe illness, those with pre-existing conditions (hypertension, pulmonary disease, diabetes, and cardiovascular disease), racial/ethnic minorities, older age, and male sex, may also be more likely to experience loneliness and social isolation [10]. Studies have suggested that COVID-19 preventive behaviors may result in greater odds of reporting loneliness and social isolation [11–13]. For instance, a population-based study in the United States (U.S.) examining the impact of COVID-19 social distancing and preventive behaviors found that 54% of participants reported loneliness [14]. Loneliness was associated with more significant depressive symptoms among people with fewer social interactions than those who had more frequent in-person social interactions or connections [14].

Given the COVID-19 pandemic and the need for continued social distancing and preventative measures, novel ways to promote social connectedness and reduce feelings of loneliness are greatly needed. New technologies have been proposed as one way to counter social distancing and stay-at-home orders while encouraging social interactions and social connectedness [15]. Studies examining COVID-19 preventive behaviors and technology use suggest that novel technologies may promote social connectedness and reduce feelings of loneliness [16,17]. However, there is a need for a theory-driven approach to aid understanding of factors associated with new technology and ways that promote the technology use to improve social connectedness during the COVID-19 pandemic.

The Multi-Theory Model (MTM) of health behavior change is a unique theory that can be utilized to explain the factors related to both initiating and sustaining new health behaviors [18]. Three constructs of MTM represent the initiation phase of behavior change, including participatory dialogue (advantages offsetting the disadvantages of the health behavior change), behavioral confidence (beliefs that one can perform the behavior change), and changes in the physical environment (having resources at one's disposal for the behavior change). Sustenance includes the following constructs: emotional transformation (translating feelings into goals for the behavior change), practice for change (creating new habits that support the health behavior change), and changes in the social environment (obtaining social support to help one maintain the health behavior change). Previous studies have shown that the MTM of health behavior change is effective in promoting and sustaining a variety of health behaviors, including handwashing, physical activity, portion sizes, consuming water instead of sugar-sweetened beverages, and potentially increasing the uptake of technology [19–23].

To our knowledge, no studies have investigated the use of MTM or related theories in promoting technology use among populations at risk for loneliness and social isolation due to the COVID-19 pandemic. This study explores the determinants of new technology use for promoting social connectedness during the COVID-19 pandemic by utilizing the conceptual paradigm of MTM. Specifically, we investigated whether the factors related to both the initiation and sustainability constructs of MTM would be associated with new technology use during the COVID-19 pandemic in a nationally representative sample of adults in the United States.

2. Materials and Methods

2.1. Study Design and Data Collection

This cross-sectional study collected data from 22 February 2021 to 25 February 2021 through Qualtrics utilizing a high-quality panel of participants. Available online: https://www.qualtrics.com/research-services/online-sample/). The general information to use Qualtrics panel platforms has been described by Miller and colleagues [24].

2.2. Eligibility Criteria:

The sample was recruited through Qualtrics to include U.S. residents aged 18 years or above with a sufficient understanding of the English language. A priori quota sampling was established to recruit a targeted sample. Quota sampling was performed to recruit a sample that mirrored Census representation by sex, race, and ethnicity. Sampling quotas for age and regional/geographical distribution were not used for sampling.

2.3. Ethical Considerations

The study (protocol # 1721549-1) was considered an exempt research study by the Institutional Review Board (IRB). Participation in the study was voluntary, and details about the study's objectives and significance were provided to participants before completing the survey. Personal identifiers were not collected to ensure anonymity. Multiple responses from the same participants were restricted by enforcing the Ballot Box Stuffing option. In other words, only one response per participant was allowed. Quality checks were performed to exclude responses completed in less than 2 min (reflective of participants not responding thoughtfully).

2.4. Data Protection and Information Security

This study utilized data obtained through a contractual agreement between the principal investigator (PI) and Qualtrics Research Services group. As an essential part of the contract, all data privacy laws and regulations were followed by both parties. Qualtrics research services do not allow the collection of any respondent's personal information. All personal identifiers were completely removed to maintain confidentiality. All electronic files of de-identified data were kept secure within the institution file storage network and regularly backed up to an encrypted and password-protected external hard drive, stored in a locked safe in a locked office of the researchers. Only researchers approved by this proposed protocol had access to the file storage network that housed these data. Desktop computers and user logins associated with this study were password-protected.

2.5. Survey Questionnaire

As guided by MTM, a 40-item survey questionnaire was developed to measure the use and acceptance of new technologies for improving social connectedness during the COVID-19 pandemic. The survey comprised 14 items related to demographic background, 3 items for social isolation, and 23 items for the two primary MTM theoretical constructs (initiation and sustenance). The face and content validity of the questionnaire was assessed by a panel of 6 subject matter experts (SMEs), who provided feedback to improve the survey. The panel review was blinded, meaning SMEs were not aware of other's input on the survey. A total of 23 changes/clarifications, primarily to improve readability, were incorporated in the instrument between rounds 1 and 2 of the SMEs' review. The questionnaire was reviewed 3 times after incorporating SMEs' feedback before dissemination of the survey. Detailed information about MTM constructs (initiation, sustenance, and social isolation) is shown in Figure 1. All constructs of initiation and sustenance were measured on a 5-point Likert scale [18]. To examine social isolation during the COVID-19 pandemic, 3 items were used to assess. The summative score of 3 social isolation items ranged from 1–12 units, and a higher score indicated more social isolation. The instrument was developed using clear and appropriate language corresponding to the Flesch reading ease of 66.0 and Flesch-Kincaid Grade Level of 6.7 grade [18,25].

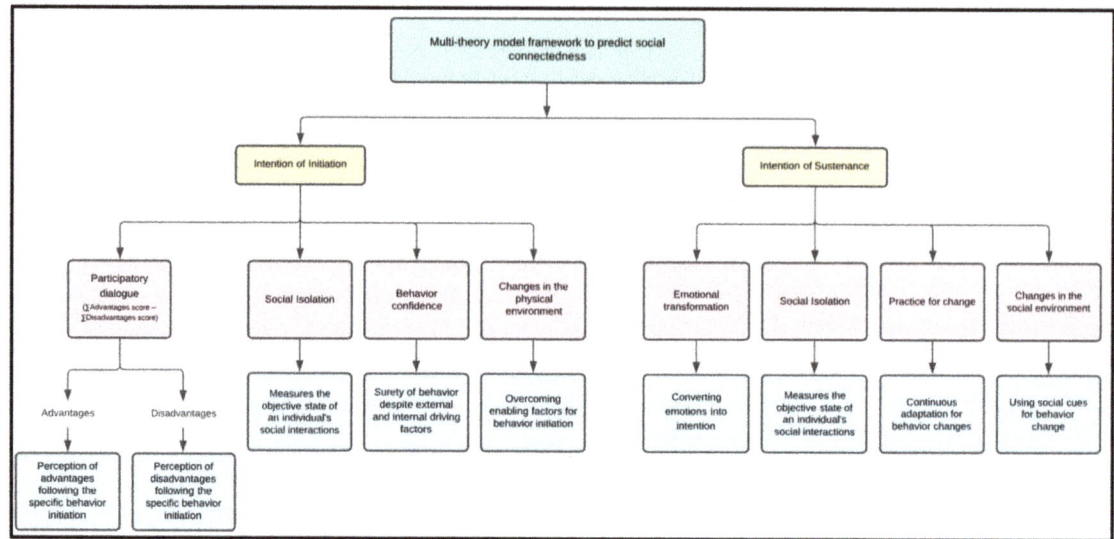

Figure 1. Flowchart detailing multi-theory model framework to predict social connectedness.

2.6. Statistical Analysis

Participants' responses to Qualtrics were exported to a spreadsheet and then imported to IBM SPSS version 27.0 (IBM Corp. Armonk, NY, USA) for analysis. Confirmatory factor analysis (CFA) using the extraction method of maximum likelihood was utilized. Reliability diagnostics or Cronbach's alpha was computed for all the subscales. Critical values for determining one-factor solution were set according to the prespecified literature's criteria [26]. The critical value for a correlation coefficient at $\alpha = 0.01$ for a 2-tailed test for the sample size of 400 participants was 0.129. This was doubled for testing the significance of loading [26]. Hence, a critical value of 0.258 was deemed appropriate [26]. The normality assumption of data was assessed using the Shapiro–Wilk test and normal Q-Q plots. An independent-samples- t-test was utilized to compare the mean scores across new technology users and non-user groups. A chi-square test was conducted to compare categorical variables. A post-hoc contingency table analysis using adjusted residuals (or Z scores) was performed in case of multiple comparisons. Bonferroni corrected p-values were generated. Bootstrapped significance testing for the chi-square test was conducted to examine replicability and consistency. The score of social isolation was dichotomized as low social isolation (≤ 6.0) and high social isolation (>6.0) by using the median-split method [27]. Categorical variables were expressed as counts and proportions, whereas continuous variables were represented as means and standard deviations. Two separate Hierarchical Regression Models (HRM) were built to predict the variance in the likelihood of initiation and sustenance of new technology behavior by multiple factors, such as demographic characteristics, social isolation, and MTM constructs. All assumptions of HRM were assessed. The significance level was set at 0.05, and 95% confidence intervals were reported wherever applicable.

2.7. Testing of HRM Assumptions

Our data meet all the 8 assumptions of HRM, which were as follows:

Assumption # 1: *The dependent variables of this study (initiation and sustenance) were measured on a continuous scale.*

Assumption # 2: *There were 2 or more independent variables, which were measured either at continuous (initiation and sustenance constructs) or nominal level (demographic variables).*

Assumption # 3: *There was a linear relationship between the continuous independent and dependent variables as assessed by partial regression plots.*

Assumption # 4: *There was independence of residual errors as assessed by a Durbin–Watson statistic.*

Assumption # 5: *No multicollinearity between the variables was assessed.*

Assumption # 6: *There were no significant outliers, as no data point was above 3 standard deviations.*

Assumption # 7: *The errors (residuals) were normally distributed, as assessed by a Q-Q plot.*

Assumption # 8: *There was homoscedasticity of residuals as assessed by visual inspection of a plot between residual versus predicted values.*

2.8. Sample Size Justification

Priori power analysis was conducted to determine sample size using G* Power statistical software. The sample sizes for independent-samples t-test and chi-square analysis were estimated depending upon Cohen's effect sizes conventions [28,29]. The total sample size estimated with a power of 0.99 was $n = 254$ for the t-test, $n = 297$ for the Chi-square test, and $n = 146$ for the regression analysis using the effect sizes of 0.5, 0.3, and 0.15, respectively. The sample size with the greatest value ($n = 297$) was considered appropriate given it satisfied the minimum requirement of all statistical tests proposed. After factoring in 25% oversampling to offset missing values, our minimum sample requirement was $n = 371$.

3. Results

Sample Characteristics

The survey was completed by a total of 382 participants. Only five responses (1.8%) were incomplete and were deleted (case-wise) from the study. Among the 382 participants, the distribution was comparable among sex categories (50.3% females vs. 49.5% males, Table 1). The mean age of the sample was 43.9 ± 18.3 years. The sample was predominantly White (71.2%, $n = 272$) and non-Hispanic (82.7%, $n = 316$; Table 1). Nearly 25% (99 of 382) of participants had a yearly income of less than $25,000. Nearly a third of participants reported being "never married" (Table 1). Of 382 participants, 202 (52.9%) used new technology during the COVID-19 pandemic, and video conferencing was the most commonly used technology in combination with other technologies. More than 50% of the sample population had a higher social isolation score indicative of loneliness (Table 1). Participants who reported new technology use were younger (<55 years of age) (73.1% vs. 26.9%; $p = 0.02$), non-Hispanic/Latino (78.9% vs. 21.1%; $p = 0.02$), employed (56.4% vs. 43.6%; $p < 0.0001$), had an income over $125,000 (12.3% vs. 3.2%; $p < 0.0001$), had health insurance (88.5% vs. 11.5%; $p < 0.0001$), were socially isolated (54.6% vs. 45.4%; $p < 0.0001$), and more likely to access smartphones with internet (Table 2).

Except for the score of disadvantages, there were significant differences in the mean scores for all constructs of initiation and sustenance among technology users and non-users (Table 3). Technology users had a statistically significant higher mean scores for initiation compared to technology non-users (2.72 ± 1.2 vs. 1.82 ± 1.3, 95% Confidence Interval [−1.151, −0.646], $p < 0.0001$, Table 3). Similarly, the mean score for sustenance was higher among technology users compared to non-users (2.78 ± 1.09 vs. 1.99 ± 1.23, 95% CI [−1.028, −0.544], $p < 0.0001$, Table 3). Participants who used new technology were more likely to report social isolation than technology non-users (M = 6.96 vs. 5.51; $p < 0.0001$ with a mean difference of 1.46 [95% CI: 0.784, 2.13].

Table 1. Descriptive statistics of the study population (n = 382).

Variable	Characteristics	Mean ± SD	n (%)
Age	-	43.9 ± 18.3	-
Sex	Female	-	192 (50.3)
	Male	-	189 (49.5)
Race	White/Caucasian	-	272 (71.2)
	Non-white	-	110 (28.8)
Ethnicity	Hispanic	-	66 (17.3)
	Non-Hispanic	-	316 (82.7)
Employment	Yes	-	177 (46.3)
	No	-	205 (53.7)
Number of hours worked weekly * Income	-	36.1 ± 25.3	-
	<$25,000	-	99 (25.9)
	$25,001–$50,000	-	92 (24.1)
	$50,001–$75,000	-	77 (20.2)
	$75,001–$100,000	-	37 (9.7)
	$100,001–$125,000	-	24 (6.3)
	>$125,000	-	33 (8.7)
	Prefer not to answer	-	20 (5.2)
Residence	Rural	-	111 (29.1)
	Semiurban	-	129 (33.8)
	Urban	-	142 (37.1)
Health insurance	Yes	-	325 (85.1)
	No	-	57 (14.9)
Marital status	Married	-	170 (44.5)
	Never married	-	117 (30.6)
	Divorced/separated	-	43 (11.3)
	Widowed	-	16 (4.2)
	Others **	-	36 (9.4)
Smartphone with internet	Yes	-	357 (93.5)
	No	-	25 (6.5)
Used new technology during COVID-19	Yes	-	227 (59.4)
	No	-	155 (40.6)
Social isolation	Low (score ≤6.0)	-	202 (52.9)
	High (score > 6.0)	-	180 (47.1)
Type of technology used	Video conferencing	-	48 (12.6)
	Smartphone apps	-	36 (9.4)
	M-health	-	11 (2.9)
	Other ***	-	33 (8.7)
	More than one (the combination of the above)	-	155 (40.6)
	None	-	99 (25.9)
Mobile phone	Yes	-	365 (95.5)
	No	-	17 (4.5)

* Number of hours were reported by 169 (44.2%) participants only. ** Other categories include a member of unmarried couple+ registered domestic partnership. *** Other categories in a type of technology include Virtual reality, video games, social sharing platforms, and exergames.

Table 2. Comparison of categories across technology users and non-users, (*n* = 382).

Variable	Characteristics	New Technology Use During COVID-19 n (%)		p-Value
		(Yes, n = 227, 59.4%)	(No, n = 155, 40.6%)	
Age groups	<55 years	166 (73.1)	95 (61.3)	0.02
	≥55 years	61 (26.9)	60 (38.7)	-
Sex	Female	119 (52.4)	73 (47.1)	0.4
	Male	107 (47.1)	82 (52.9)	-
Race	White/Caucasian	162 (71.4)	110 (71.0)	0.9
	Non-white	65 (28.6)	45 (29.0)	-
Ethnicity	Hispanic	48 (21.1)	18 (11.6)	0.02
	Non-Hispanic	179 (78.9)	137 (88.4)	-
Employment	Yes	128 (56.4)	49 (31.6)	<0.0001
	No	99 (43.6)	106 (68.4)	-
Income	<$25,000	43 (18.9)	56 (36.1)	<0.0001 *
	$25,001–$50,000	52 (22.9)	40 (25.8)	0.5
	$50,001–$75,000	51 (22.5)	26 (16.8)	0.2
	$75,001–$100,000	23 (10.1)	14 (9.0)	0.7
	$100,001–$125,000	20 (8.8)	4 (2.6)	0.6
	>$125,000	28 (12.3)	5 (3.2)	<0.0001 *
Residence	Rural	58 (25.6)	53 (34.2)	0.1
	Semiurban	77 (33.9)	52 (33.5)	-
	Urban	92 (40.5)	50 (32.3)	-
Health insurance	Yes	201 (88.5)	124 (80.0)	0.02
	No	26 (11.5)	31 (20.0)	-
Marital status	Married	106 (46.7)	64 (41.3)	0.5
	Never married	69 (30.4)	48 (31.0)	-
	Divorced/Separated	21 (9.3)	22 (14.2)	-
	Widowed	8 (3.5)	8 (5.2)	-
	Others	23 (10.1)	13 (8.4)	-
Social isolation	Low (score ≤ 6.0)	103 (45.4)	99 (63.9)	<0.0001
	High (score > 6.0)	124 (54.6)	56 (36.1)	-
Smartphone with internet	Yes	219 (96.5)	138 (89.0)	0.004
	No	8 (3.5)	17 (11.0)	-
Mobile phone	Yes	223 (98.2)	142 (91.6)	0.002
	No	4 (1.8)	13 (8.4)	-

* *p*-values in multiple comparisons are Bonferroni corrected.

Two separate hierarchical multiple regression models were utilized to predict the variance in initiation and sustenance of the behavior by MTM constructs beyond demographic variables among technology users and non-users (Table 4). Among participants using technology during a pandemic, the full model (Model 4) to predict initiation was statistically significant, $R^2 = 0.408$, F (9216) = 16.545, $p < 0.0001$; adjusted $R^2 = 0.383$ (Table 4). All MTM constructs added statistical significance to the prediction. The standardized regression coefficient value indicated that the behavior confidence was associated with the maximum increase of 0.455 points on the initiation score (Table 4). Similarly, for sustenance model, the Model 4 was statistically significant and improved prediction, $R^2 = 0.449$, $F (9216) = 19.546$, $p < 0.0001$; adjusted $R^2 = 0.426$ (Table 4). The value of the standardized regression coefficient in the sustenance model indicated that the emotional transformation was associated with the maximum increase of 0.326 points on the initiation score among technology users (Table 4).

Table 3. Comparing mean scores of MTM constructs and reliability diagnostics across groups.

Groups	Those Who Used Technology During COVID-19 ($n = 227$)				Those Who Did Not Use Technology During COVID-19 ($n = 155$)				
Constructs	Possible Score Range	Observed Score Range	Mean ± SD	Cronbach's Alpha	Possible Score Range	Observed Score Range	Mean ± SD	Cronbach's Alpha	p-Value *
Initiation	0–4	0–4	2.72± 1.2	-	0–4	0–4	1.82 ± 1.3	-	<0.0001
Social isolation	0–12	0–12	6.96 ± 3.0	0.83	0–12	0–12	5.51 ± 3.6	0.83	<0.0001
Participatory dialogue: advantages	0–12	0–12	7.16 ± 2.79	0.83	0–12	0–12	4.77 ± 3.3	0.90	<0.0001
Participatory dialogue: disadvantages	0–12	0–12	4.68 ± 3.11	0.79	0–12	0–12	4.68 ± 3.13	0.77	0.9
Participatory dialogue **	−12–+12	−8–+12	2.48 ± 3.4	-	−12–+12	−12–+10	0.09 ± 3.8	-	<0.0001
Behavior confidence	0–12	0–12	8.25± 2.87	0.81	0–12	0–12	6.48 ± 3.4	0.87	<0.0001
Changes in the physical environment	0–12	0–12	7.61 ± 3.1	0.81	0–12	0–12	5.72 ± 3.5	0.86	<0.0001
Entire initiation scale	-	-	-	0.82	-	-	-	0.84	-
Sustenance	0–4	0–4	2.78 ± 1.09	-	0–4	0–4	1.99 ± 1.23	-	<0.0001
Emotional transformation	0–12	0–12	7.48± 3.05	0.85	0–12	0–12	5.63 ± 3.45	0.89	<0.0001
Practice for change	0–12	0–12	7.43 ± 3.04	0.83	0–12	0–12	5.80 ± 3.58	0.90	<0.0001
Changes in the social environment	0–12	0–12	7.49 ± 2.98	0.73	0–12	0–12	5.75 ± 3.46	0.81	<0.0001
Entire sustenance scale	-	-	-	0.90	-	-	-	0.94	-
Entire scale	-	-	-	0.91	-	-	-	0.93	-

* p-values of independent-samples-t test ** participatory dialogue (advantages-disadvantages).

Table 4. Predicting likelihood for initiation and sustenance of technology users ($n = 227$) through HRM.

Variables	Model 1		Model 2		Model 3		Model 4	
	B	β	B	β	B	β	B	β
The Likelihood for Initiation as a Dependent Variable								
Constant	2.34 **	-	2.23 **	-	1.22 **	-	0.59	-
Age	−0.074	−0.028	−0.176	−0.067	−0.015	−0.006	−0.016	−0.006
Sex	−0.130	−0.056	−0.107	−0.046	−0.155	−0.067	−0.140	−0.060
Income	0.054	0.083	0.059	0.090	−0.012	−0.019	0.003	0.005
Social isolation	0.056	0.146	0.046	0.119	0.023	0.059	0.017	0.043
Participatory dialogue	-	-	0.105 **	0.307	0.056 **	0.163	0.054 *	0.158
Changes in the physical environment	-	-	-	-	0.176 **	0.472	0.053 *	0.143
Behavioral confidence	-	-	-	-	-	-	0.184 **	0.455
R^2	0.038	-	0.130	-	0.310	-	0.408	-
F	1.43	-	4.64 **	-	12.19 **	-	16.55 **	-

Table 4. Cont.

Variables	Model 1		Model 2		Model 3		Model 4	
ΔR^2	0.038	-	0.092	-	0.180	-	0.098	-
ΔF^2	1.43	-	23.03 **	-	56.75 **	-	35.74 **	-
The Likelihood for Sustenance as a Dependent Variable								
Constant	2.51 **	-	1.12 **	-	0.94 **	-	0.80 **	-
Age	−0.011	−0.005	0.059	0.024	0.122	0.050	0.167	0.069
Sex	−0.161	−0.075	−0.153	−0.071	−0.165	−0.076	−0.161	−0.074
Income	0.035	0.059	0.005	0.008	−0.003	−0.005	−0.017	−0.027
Social isolation	0.029	0.082	−0.005	−0.014	−0.005	−0.014	−0.012	−0.032
Emotional transformation	-	-	0.218 **	0.619	0.138 **	0.390	0.115 **	0.326
Practice for change	-	-	-	-	0.100 **	0.282	0.086 **	0.243
Changes in the social environment	-	-	-	-	-	-	0.061 *	0.169
R^2	0.040	-	0.408	-	0.433	-	0.449	-
F	1.507	-	21.46 **	-	20.68 **	-	19.55 **	-
ΔR^2	0.040	-	0.368	-	0.025	-	0.016	-
ΔF^2	1.507	-	135.64 **	-	9.40 **	-	6.389 *	-

B (Unstandardized coefficient); β (Standardized coefficient), * p-value < 0.05; ** p-value < 0.001.

Among participants not using new technology during the pandemic (Model 4), initiation was statistically significant, R^2 = 0.430, F (9, 145) = 12.178, p < 0.0001; adjusted R^2 = 0.395 (Table 5). In addition, in a regression analysis with sustenance as a dependent variable, the full model (Model 4) was statistically significant, R^2 = 0.513, F (9, 145) = 16.941, p < 0.0001; adjusted R^2 = 0.482 (Table 5). The value of standardized regression coefficients indicated that the changes in the physical environment were associated with an increase of 0.300 units on the initiation score among technology non-users (Table 5). Regarding sustenance, changes in the social environment were associated with an increase of 0.393 units in the sustenance among technology non-users (Table 5).

A confirmatory factor analysis (CFA) was performed on eight theoretical constructs (7 MTM construct and 1 social isolation) to establish construct validity of the subscales. The suitability of CFA was assessed before the analysis. Bartlett's Test of Sphericity was statistically significant (p < 0.0005), indicating that the data were likely factorizable. Inspection of the correlation matrix indicated that all variables had at least one correlation coefficient greater than 0.3. The overall Kaiser–Meyer–Olkin (KMO) measure was 0.87, which classifies as "middling" to "meritorious", according to Kaiser [30]. CFA revealed that all MTM constructs (advantages, disadvantages, behavior confidence, changes in the physical environment, emotional transformation, practice for change, changes in the social environment, and construct of social isolation met Eigenvalue-one criteria and explained 71.0%, 54.5%, 66.0%, 65.0%, 71.0%, 69.4%, 56.0%, and 65.2% of the total variance, respectively. All subscales had a one-factor solution, and all factor loadings were more than twice the critical value of 0.28 [31]. The minimum factor loading was 0.643.

Table 5. Predicting likelihood for initiation and sustenance of technology non-users (n = 155) through HRM.

Variables	Model 1		Model 2		Model 3		Model 4	
	B	β	B	β	B	β	B	β
The Likelihood For Initiation As A Dependent Variable								
Constant	1.965 **	-	1.899 **	-	0.909 *	-	0.596	-
Age	−0.466 *	−0.179	−0.450*	−0.172	−0.317	−0.121	−0.286	−0.110
Sex	0.459 *	0.180	0.567 **	0.222	0.358 *	0.140	0.372 *	0.146
Income	0.066	0.090	0.063	0.085	0.025	0.035	0.036	0.049
Social isolation	0.033	0.095	0.021	0.059	−0.009	−0.027	−0.005	−0.014
Participatory dialogue	-	-	0.099 **	0.030	0.051 *	0.154	0.039	0.117
Changes in the physical environment	-	-	-	-	0.190 **	0.526	0.109 **	0.300
Behavioral confidence	-	-	-	-	-	-	0.109 **	0.293
R^2	0.083	-	0.166	-	0.400	-	0.430	-
F	2.23 *	-	4.18 **	-	12.17 **	-	12.18 **	-
ΔR^2	0.083	-	0.083	-	0.234	-	0.030	-
ΔF^2	2.23 *	-	14.61 **	-	56.99 **	-	7.76 **	-
The likelihood for Sustenance as a dependent variable								
Constant	1.639 **	-	0.092	-	0.052	-	0.006	-
Age	−0.221	−0.087	0.103	0.041	0.079	0.031	0.030	0.012
Sex	0.443 *	0.180	0.288	0.117	0.311	0.126	0.323 *	0.131
Income	0.018	0.025	−0.023	−0.033	−0.026	−0.037	−0.041	−0.058
Social isolation	0.072 **	0.211	0.057 *	0.167	0.54 *	0.159 *	0.048	0.141
Emotional transformation	-	-	0.215 **	0.602	0.106 *	0.295	0.052	0.144
Practice for change	-	-	-	-	0.117 *	0.341	0.072	0.208
Changes in the social environment	-	-	-	-	-	-	0.140 **	0.393
R^2	0.092	-	0.417	-	0.439	-	0.513	-
F	2.495 *	-	15.05 **	-	14.3 **	-	16.94 **	-
ΔR^2	0.092	-	0.326	-	0.021	-	0.074	-
ΔF^2	2.50 *	-	82.5 **	-	5.55 *	-	21.94 **	-

* p-value < 0.05; ** p-value < 0.001.

4. Discussion

The purpose of this study was to assess the determinants of new technology adoption to promote social connectedness during the COVID-19 pandemic utilizing the conceptual paradigm of MTM. The scientific value of this research lies in its contribution to building evidence-based or theory-based support for developing putative interventions to build social connectedness in the COVID-19 pandemic. As expected, all the three initiation constructs of MTM (participatory dialogue, changes in the physical environment, and behavioral confidence) were statistically significant predictors of the likelihood of initiating new technology use among technology users. These accounted for 38.3% of the variance. Similarly, all the three sustenance constructs of MTM (practice for change, emotional transformation, and changes in the social environment) were statistically significant predictors of the likelihood of continuing new technology use among technology users and accounted for 42.6% of the variance. These findings confirm that the MTM constructs help understand both starting and continuing the use of technology during the COVID-19 pandemic in a nationally representative sample of the population. Our findings reached substantial explanatory power in the behavioral and social sciences [25]. There can be other potential factors that contribute to the performance of any behavior, such as genetics, personality characteristics, irrational beliefs, social norms, policies, etc., that cannot be measured in any given study, thus preventing accountability of predictability to close to 100%. The findings are further supported by modeling conducted with non-technology users in which behavioral confidence and changes in the physical environment were significant contributors along with sex for starting the use of the new technology and accounted for 39.5% of the variance. These were indicative of a positive association in consonance with the theoretical proposition. Similarly, changes in the social environment and sex were significant, accounting for 48.2% of the variance and indicative of a positive association per the theoretical proposition. These findings among non-technology users combined with the findings mentioned above with technology users, lend credibility to MTM as a strong explanatory model on which interventions to promote technology use can be designed. All the constructs of MTM are modifiable, making it easy to translate them into intervention designing and evaluation.

The study also found that social isolation (6.24 ± 3.3) was a problem during the COVID-19 pandemic. While the sample size was limited, a total of 47.1% of the respondents reported having high levels of social isolation (score above 6.0 units on a scale of 0–12). These findings were consistent with reports from Rosenberg and colleagues (2020) that the prevalence of loneliness was 54% during the COVID-19 pandemic in April 2020 [14]. Our study was conducted in March 2021 when restrictions were relatively relaxed, resulting in slightly lower rates of social isolation. While social isolation has been reported as a significant problem during the COVID-19 pandemic [5,12,31], and the use of technology has been suggested as a means to cope with it [15,32,33]. We could not find any systematic studies that linked the use of technology with social isolation or loneliness during the COVID-19 pandemic. Prior to the COVID-19 pandemic, the problem of social isolation and loneliness was still relatively high and was known to have adverse health consequences [34]. Nearly half the population in our sample reported that social isolation was a problem, which underscores the need for rigorous public health efforts. The promotion of new technology can serve as an effective tool in the repertoire of public health professionals. The COVID-19 pandemic has provided an impetus for the promotion of new technology, which should be channeled into future intervention planning.

Regarding the use of new technology, it was found that 40.6% have not used any new technology. This is especially relevant because 93.5% of participants had reported current access to a smartphone with the internet, and 95.5% owned a mobile phone. Smartphones can be used as potent means to promote interventions in the future. Furthermore, this study found a higher mean score of social isolation among technology users than non-technology users. This may be due to a high degree of socially isolated individuals in this group being more motivated to use new technology to connect with others. Our study examined the following types of new technology use: video conferencing, smartphone apps, mHealth, virtual reality, video games, social sharing platforms, and exergames. Since the questionnaire asked the respondents to mark all the options they were using, 40.7% of respondents marked more than one category, followed by the use of video-conferencing alone (12.6%).

A closer examination of each construct of MTM guides health promotion program planning to address social isolation and the role of new technology use. In the initiation model, the construct of behavioral confidence had the largest and statistically significant contribution for technology users and non-technology users, indicating it to be the strongest predictor. This finding is supported by several studies, for example, Yoshany and colleagues (2021) found behavioral confidence to be a significant and strongest predictor in their study of nutritional behaviors among menopausal women [35]. Sharma and colleagues, in their study predicting handwashing behavior, found a significant and strongest behavioral confidence construct in the study sample [21]. Williams and colleagues also found a significant and strongest contribution of behavioral confidence for changes in fruit and vegetable consumption behavior among Black men [36]. Our findings suggest that behavioral confidence must be developed among the general population to use new technology during the COVID-19 and post-pandemic periods to improve social connectedness and reduce social isolation and loneliness. Behavioral confidence can be built in interventions promoting new technology by introducing the learning into small steps, using multiple internal and external sources that infuse confidence, projecting acquisition of behavior change to a future date, and reducing associated stress.

The second construct found to be important in our study for starting the adoption of new technology to improve social connectedness was physical environment changes that entail accessibility and availability of newer technology. This finding is also supported by other studies on MTM with the availability of fruits and vegetables [36] and healthy nutritional options [35]. The construct also aligns with the diffusion of innovations theory construct involving adopting innovations [36,37]. With technology innovations, various environmental factors such as reducing complexity, increasing compatibility, improving demonstrability, reducing costs, and allowing for modifications by the user may be useful aspects to keep in mind for interventions promoting new technology, especially among those experiencing social isolation [23,38].

The construct of participatory dialogue (e.g., the participant is convinced that the positives of using new technology outweigh the negatives of using new technology) was significant for technology users but not for non-technology users. This finding underscores the need for designing interventions that promote the positives aspects of new technology to enhance its adoption among potential users. This finding is also supported by the construct of the relative advantage, or how new technology may appear to be better than other alternatives, as advocated in Roger's diffusion of innovations theory [37]. Other constructs from this model such as compatibility, reduction of complexity, demonstrability, reduction of costs, and clarity of results may also be important aspects to highlight during participatory dialogue.

For continued use of new technology, the construct of changes in the social environment in MTM was statistically significant for both technology users and non-technology users. The higher values of estimated coefficients indicate the need for continued social support to maintain putative behavior change among non-users. This construct is important in several studies, which tested the applicability of MTM. For example, studies have found that changes in the social environment were important for physical activity behavior change [39], portion size behavior change [22], and fruit and vegetable consumption behavior change [40]. This construct is also important from the perspective of diffusion of innovations theory that emphasizes the construct of the social system. Social networks, change agents, opinion leaders, and person-to-person dissemination are important for adopting innovations such as new technology [37].

The construct of emotional transformation in MTM or directing feelings towards using new technology to connect with others was significant for technology users ($\beta = 0.326$, $p < 0.001$) but not for non-technology users. The recognition and regulation of emotions is an essential part of emotional intelligence [41]. This concept is gaining popularity and could be pivotal for promoting the use of technology for social connectedness. In several applications of MTM, this construct has demonstrated significance regarding physical activity behavior change [39], portion size behavior changes [22], and replacing sugar-sweetened beverage consumption with water [42]. The negative emotions of sadness, helplessness, despair, feeling stressed, feeling anxious, and so on can all be channeled into positive applications of applying energy toward learning and using technology to connect with others, especially during the COVID-19 pandemic.

The construct of practice for change in MTM or persistent thinking about using technology to connect with others was significant for technology users ($\beta = 0.243$, $p < 0.001$) but not for non-technology users. This construct facilitates the initial adoption of new technology and then supports its continued use [18,23]. In several MTM based studies, this construct is influential in explaining the maintenance of behavior change [23,39,40]. Thus, ample opportunity for practicing and reflecting on the use of technology holds promise for increasing social connectedness and reducing social isolation during the COVID-19 pandemic.

In our study, several demographic characteristics were found to be significant with technology use. For example, there was a significant difference between older and younger populations. We operationalized age as a dichotomous variable comprising those under 55 years of age and those 55 years of age and older. As expected, we found that the use of new technology was significantly lower among those over 55 years of age. Future research on identifying technology use correlations specific to older populations may be necessary for reducing social isolation during the COVID-19 pandemic. There is a need to design different interventions for younger and older populations.

Another demographic characteristic that we found to be significantly different between users and non-users of technology was ethnicity, with fewer Hispanics (21.1%) using new technology ($p = 0.02$). This finding is somewhat contrary to the findings of a study on HIV prevention among Hispanic women that found high levels of comfort with technology use [43], and also a study was performed in New York that a large majority of Hispanics had computers at home and used the internet regularly [44]. Further, as expected, 68.4% of unemployed participants were not using new technology ($p <0.0001$). This could be related to their non-affordability of new technology. Likewise, respondents earning less than $25,000 per year (36.1%) were more non-users. This could also be related to the non-affordability of new technology. There is a need to target some of these subgroups that exhibit greater disparities.

4.1. Implications for Practice

There is a need for technology promotion programs at all levels to improve social connectedness to alleviate social isolation during the COVID-19 pandemic. Such programs can be promoted by health education specialists, healthcare providers, health workers, counselors, mental health professionals, public health professionals, policymakers, computer professionals, etc. The new technology can include the utilization of m-Health (i.e., use of mobile phones as part of a health program), smartphone apps (e.g., WhatsApp, Instagram, Facetime, Skype, etc.), virtual reality in groups (e.g., guided meditation in groups using virtual assets), video conferencing (e.g., Zoom, WebEx, etc.), videogames (i.e., multi-player games), exergames using multiple users (i.e., phone or computer-based group exercise in groups), and social sharing platforms (e.g., "My Country Talks"; https://www.mycountrytalks.org) [45].

MTM serves as a useful framework in promoting new technology use. For instance, facilitating behavior change is part of behavioral confidence, which can be built by exploring the sources for enhancing the ability to use technology that appeals to the person. This can come in the form of letting users experiment with newer technology, having YouTube tutorial guides, providing short and simple stepwise guides both online and in technology. Secondly, changes in the physical environment in the form of new technology availability are also important for starting the adoption of new technology. Subsidizing availability, especially for individuals from lower-income backgrounds, should be a priority for policy action.

For the continuation of the use of new technology also MTM constructs can help. The construct of changes in the social environment helps to explain the fostering of social networks, utilizing change agents, mobilizing opinion leaders, and using friends and family members can serve as effective means to promote the continued use of new technology. In previous interventions of MTM, changes in social environment construct have been used to promote behavior change and foster the use of technology [19,46]. The constructs of emotional transformation whereby directing negative feelings into positive ones for the use of technology and practice for change of constant practice of new technology will also go a long way in improving the continued use of technology.

4.2. Strengths and Limitations

To our knowledge, this is the first study that looks at theory-based correlates of the use of new technology in the COVID-19 pandemic to improve social connectedness. The study provides evidence that social isolation is becoming a problem in modern times, and new technology can help in this process. The study provides a psychometrically robust instrument that can be used for testing future intervention applications. The utilization of an up-to-date model such as MTM can help in adopting new technology. There are also several limitations of the study. A cross-sectional study limits the establishment of causal inferences due to data on independent correlations and dependent variables being collected simultaneously. Further, reliance on self-reports introduces potential measurement bias. Next, there can be other potential factors, including genetics, personality characteristics, irrational beliefs, social norms, policies, which may affect the performance of the behavior change and cannot be measured in any given study. These unmeasured variables may prevent accountability of predictability to close to 100%. Finally, even though we collected data from a nationally representative sample in terms of gender and race, all other variables, including age and region/geographical distribution, could have introduced sampling bias, which limits the generalizability of our findings. Moreover, the sole purpose of this study was model testing and did not determine the prevalence estimates. Moreover, COVID-19 restrictions posed challenges in the sampling. Future studies with a relatively bigger sample size can be planned to estimate prevalence.

5. Conclusions

During the COVID-19 pandemic, social isolation has grown, and there is a need to improve social connectedness through new technology. The study provides evidence that MTM is a useful model in explaining the promotion and adoption of new technology to address the issue of social isolation and promoting social connectedness. Future research should discern the determinants of social connectedness based on MTM for various subgroups based on factors such as age, race/ethnicity, employment status, etc. There is an ardent need to design and test the efficacy of interventions based on MTM that can be utilized to promote social connectedness through the use of new technology. In summary, MTM can lead the way for evidence-based intervention planning in this regard.

Author Contributions: Conceptualization, M.S. and K.B.; methodology, K.B.; software, K.B.; validation, M.S., K.B., and J.F.; formal analysis, K.B.; investigation, K.B.; resources, M.S. and K.B.; data curation, M.S.; writing—M.S., K.B., and J.F.; writing—review and editing, M.S., K.B., and J.F.; visualization, K.B.; supervision, M.S.; project administration, K.B. All authors have read and agreed to the published version of the manuscript.

Funding: This study received funding from the School of Public Health, University of Nevada, Las Vegas for the data collection.

Institutional Review Board Statement: The study was conducted according to the guidelines of the Declaration of Helsinki and approved by the Institutional Review Board (or Ethics Committee) of the University of Nevada, Las Vegas (1721549-1 dated 18 February 2021).

Informed Consent Statement: Informed consent was obtained from all subjects involved in the study.

Data Availability Statement: The data presented in this study are available on request from the corresponding author. The data are not publicly available due to ethical reasons.

Acknowledgments: We would like to acknowledge Ravi Batra for his assistance in formatting.

Conflicts of Interest: The authors declare no conflict of interest.

References

1. Gerst-Emerson, K.; Jayawardhana, J. Loneliness as a public health issue: The impact of loneliness on health care utilization among older adults. *Am. J. Public Health* **2015**, *105*, 1013–1019. [CrossRef]
2. Jeste, D.V.; Lee, E.E.; Cacioppo, S. Battling the Modern Behavioral Epidemic of Loneliness: Suggestions for Research and Interventions. *JAMA Psychiatry* **2020**, *77*, 553–554. [CrossRef] [PubMed]
3. Murthy, V. The Surgeon General's Prescription of Happiness. *TEDMED* **2016**. Available online: https://tedmed.com/talks/show?id=527633 (accessed on 31 January 2021).
4. Cacioppo, J.T.; Cacioppo, S. The growing problem of loneliness. *Lancet* **2018**, *391*, 426. [CrossRef]
5. Hwang, T.J.; Rabheru, K.; Peisah, C.; Reichman, W.; Ikeda, M. Loneliness and social isolation during the COVID-19 pandemic. *Int. Psychogeriatr.* **2020**, *32*, 1217–1220. [CrossRef] [PubMed]

6. Chen, Y.; Feeley, T.H. Social support, social strain, loneliness, and well-being among older adults: An analysis of the Health and Retirement Study. *J. Soc. Pers. Relatsh.* **2014**, *31*, 141–161. [CrossRef]
7. Holt-Lunstad, J.; Smith, T.B.; Baker, M.; Harris, T.; Stephenson, D. Loneliness and social isolation as risk factors for mortality: A meta-analytic review. *Perspect. Psychol. Sci.* **2015**, *10*, 227–237. [CrossRef]
8. Valtorta, N.K.; Kanaan, M.; Gilbody, S.; Ronzi, S.; Hanratty, B. Loneliness and social isolation as risk factors for coronary heart disease and stroke: Systematic review and meta-analysis of longitudinal observational studies. *Heart* **2016**, *102*, 1009–1016. [CrossRef]
9. Ebinger, J.E.; Achamallah, N.; Ji, H.; Claggett, B.L.; Sun, N.; Botting, P.; Nguyen, T.; Luong, E.; Kim, E.H.; Park, E.; et al. Pre-existing traits associated with Covid-19 illness severity. *PLoS ONE* **2020**, *15*, e0236240. [CrossRef]
10. Stickley, A.; Koyanagi, A. Physical multimorbidity and loneliness: A population-based study. *PLoS ONE* **2018**, *13*, e0191651. [CrossRef]
11. Choi, E.Y.; Farina, M.P.; Wu, Q.; Ailshire, J. COVID-19 social distancing measures and loneliness among older adults. *J. Gerontol. B Psychol. Sci. Soc. Sci.* **2021**, gbab009. [CrossRef]
12. Miller, E.D. Loneliness in the era of COVID-19. *Front. Psychol.* **2020**, *11*, 1–3. [CrossRef] [PubMed]
13. Stickley, A.; Matsubayashi, T.; Ueda, M. Loneliness and COVID-19 preventive behaviours among Japanese adults. *J. Public Health* **2020**. epub ahead of print. [CrossRef] [PubMed]
14. Rosenberg, M.; Luetke, M.; Hensel, D.; Kianersi, S.; Fu, T.C.; Herbenick, D. Depression and loneliness during April 2020 COVID-19 restrictions in the United States, and their associations with frequency of social and sexual connections. *Soc. Psychiatry Psychiatr. Epidemiol.* **2021**, 1–12, epub ahead of print.
15. Shah, S.G.S.; Nogueras, D.; van Woerden, H.C.; Kiparoglou, V. The COVID-19 pandemic: A pandemic of lockdown loneliness and the role of digital technology. *J. Med. Internet Res.* **2020**, *22*, e22287. [CrossRef] [PubMed]
16. Bastoni, S.; Wrede, C.; Ammar, A.; Braakman-Jansen, A.; Sanderman, R.; Gaggioli, A.; Trabelsi, K.; Masmoudi, L.; Boukhris, O.; Glenn, J.M.; et al. Psychosocial effects and use of communication technologies during home confinement in the first wave of the COVID-19 pandemic in Italy and The Netherlands. *Int. J. Environ. Res. Public Health* **2021**, *18*, 2619. [CrossRef]
17. David, M.E.; Roberts, J.A. Smartphone use during the COVID-19 pandemic: Social versus physical distancing. *Int. J. Environ. Res. Public Health* **2021**, *18*, 1034. [CrossRef] [PubMed]
18. Sharma, M. Multi-theory model (MTM) for health behavior change. *WebmedCentral Behav.* **2015**, *6*, WMC004982.
19. Hayes, T.; Sharma, M.; Shahbazi, M.; Sung, J.H.; Bennett, R.; Reese-Smith, J. The evaluation of a fourth-generation multi-theory model (MTM) based intervention to initiate and sustain physical activity in African American women. *Health Promot. Perspect.* **2019**, *9*, 13–23. [CrossRef]
20. Batra, K.; Morgan, A.E.; Sharma, M. COVID-19 and social isolation endangering psychological health of older adults: Implications for telepsychiatry. *Signa Vitae* **2020**, *16*, 14–19.
21. Sharma, M.; Batra, K.; Davis, R.; Wilkerson, A. Explaining handwashing behavior among college students during COVID-19 pandemic using the multi-theory model (MTM) of health behavior change. *Healthcare* **2021**, *9*, 55. [CrossRef]
22. Sharma, M.; Catalano, H.P.; Nahar, V.K.; Lingam, V.; Johnson, P.; Ford, M.A. Using multi-theory model of health behavior change to predict portion size consumption among college students. *Health Promot. Perspect.* **2016**, *6*, 137–144. [CrossRef]
23. Sharma, M. *Theoretical Foundations of Health Education and Health Promotion*, 3rd ed.; Jones and Bartlett: Burlington, MA, USA, 2017; pp. 250–262.
24. Miller, C.A.; Guidry, J.P.D.; Dahman, B.; Thomson, M.D. A tale of two diverse Qualtrics samples: Information for online survey researchers. *Cancer Epidemiol. Biomark. Prev.* **2020**, *29*, 731–735. [CrossRef] [PubMed]
25. Sharma, M.; Petosa, R.L. *Measurement and Evaluation for Health Educators*, 1st ed.; Jones & Bartlett Learning: Burlington, MA, USA, 2014.
26. Kaiser, H.F. The application of electronic computers to factor Analysis. *Educ. Psychol. Meas.* **1960**, *20*, 141–151. [CrossRef]
27. DeCoster, J.; Gallucci, M.; Iselin, A.R. Best practices for using median splits, artificial categorization, and their continuous alternatives. *J. Exp. Psychopathol.* **2011**, *2*, 197–209. [CrossRef]
28. Cohen, J. *Statistical Power Analysis for the Behavioral Sciences*, 2nd ed. 1988. Available online: http://utstat.toronto.edu/~{}brunner/oldclass/378f16/readings/CohenPower.pdf (accessed on 1 February 2021).
29. Faul, F.; Erdfelder, E.; Buchner, A.; Lang, A.G. Statistical power analyses using G*Power 3.1: Tests for correlation and regression analyses. *Behav. Res. Methods* **2009**, *41*, 1149–1160. [CrossRef] [PubMed]
30. Kaiser, H.F. An index of factorial simplicity. *Psychometrika* **1974**, *39*, 32–36. [CrossRef]
31. Stevens, J. *Applied Multivariate Statistics for the Social Sciences*, 3rd ed.; Lawrence Erlbaum Associates: Mahwah, NJ, USA, 1996.
32. Banerjee, D.; Rai, M. Social isolation in Covid-19: The impact of loneliness. *Int. J. Soc. Psychiatry* **2020**, *66*, 525–527. [CrossRef] [PubMed]
33. Eghtesadi, M. Breaking social isolation amidst COVID-19: A viewpoint on improving access to technology in long-term care facilities. *J. Am. Geriatr. Soc.* **2020**, *68*, 949–950. [CrossRef] [PubMed]
34. Leigh-Hunt, N.; Bagguley, D.; Bash, K.; Turner, V.; Turnbull, S.; Valtorta, N.; Caan, W. An overview of systematic reviews on the public health consequences of social isolation and loneliness. *Public Health* **2017**, *152*, 157–171. [CrossRef]
35. Yoshany, N.; Sharma, M.; Bahri, N.; Jambarsang, S.; Morowatisharifabad, M.A. Predictors in initiating and maintaining nutritional behaviors to deal with menopausal symptoms based on multi-theory model. *Int. Q. Community Health Educ.* **2021**, 1–8. [CrossRef]

36. Williams, J.L.; Sharma, M.; Mendy, V.L.; Leggett, S.; Akil, L.; Perkins, S. Using multi theory model (MTM) of health behavior change to explain intention for initiation and sustenance of the consumption of fruits and vegetables among African American men from barbershops in Mississippi. *Health Promot. Perspect.* **2020**, *10*, 200–206. [CrossRef] [PubMed]
37. Rogers, E.M. *Diffusion of Innovations*, 5th ed.; Free Press: New York, NY, USA, 2003.
38. Greenhalgh, T.; Robert, G.; Bate, P.; Macfralane, F.; Kyriakidou, O. *Diffusion of Innovations in Health Service Organizations: A Systematic Literature Review*; Blackwell: Malden, MA, USA, 2005.
39. Nahar, V.K.; Sharma, M.; Catalano, H.P.; Ickes, M.J.; Johnson, P.; Ford, M.A. Testing multi-theory model (MTM) in predicting initiation and sustenance of physical activity behavior among college students. *Health Promot. Perspect.* **2016**, *6*, 58–65. [CrossRef] [PubMed]
40. Sharma, M.; Stephens, P.M.; Nahar, V.K.; Catalano, H.P.; Lingam, V.; Ford, M.A. Using multi-theory model to predict initiation and sustenance of fruit and vegetable consumption among college students. *J. Am. Osteopath Assoc.* **2018**, *118*, 507–517.
41. Goleman, D. *Emotional Intelligence*; Bantam: New York, NY, USA, 1995.
42. Sharma, M.; Catalano, H.P.; Nahar, V.K.; Lingam, V.; Johnson, P.; Ford, M.A. Using multi-theory model (MTM) of health behavior change to predict water consumption instead of sugar sweetened beverages. *J. Res. Health Sci.* **2017**, *17*, e00370.
43. Villegas, N.; Cianelli, R.; de Tantillo, L.; Warheit, M.; Montano, N.P.; Ferrer, L.; Patel, S. Assessment of technology use and technology preferences for HIV prevention among Hispanic women. *Hisp. Health Care Int.* **2018**, *16*, 197–203. [CrossRef]
44. Manganello, J.A.; Gerstner, G.; Pergolino, K.; Graham, Y.; Strogatz, D. Media and technology use among Hispanics/Latinos in New York: Implications for health communication programs. *J. Racial Ethn Health Disparities* **2016**, *3*, 508–517. [CrossRef] [PubMed]
45. Riva, G.; Mantovani, F.; Wiederhold, B.K. Positive technology and COVID-19. *Cyberpsychol. Behav. Soc. Netw.* **2020**, *23*, 581–587. [CrossRef]
46. Brown, L.; Sharma, M.; Leggett, S.; Sung, J.H.; Bennett, R.L.; Azevedo, M. Efficacy testing of the SAVOR (Sisters Adding Fruits and Vegetables for Optimal Results) intervention among African American women: A randomized controlled trial. *Health Promot. Perspect.* **2020**, *10*, 270–280. [CrossRef] [PubMed]

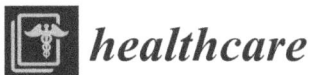

Article

Forecasting COVID-19 Confirmed Cases Using Empirical Data Analysis in Korea

Da Hye Lee [1], Youn Su Kim [1], Young Youp Koh [2], Kwang Yoon Song [1,*] and In Hong Chang [1,*]

[1] Department of Computer Science and Statistics, Chosun University, Gwangju 61452, Korea; is_hye@chosun.kr (D.H.L.); imk92315@naver.com (Y.S.K.)
[2] Department of Internal Medicine, College of Medicine and Medical School, Chosun University, Gwangju 61452, Korea; yykoh@chosun.ac.kr
* Correspondence: csssig@chosun.ac.kr (K.Y.S.); ihchang@chosun.ac.kr (I.H.C.)

Abstract: From November to December 2020, the third wave of COVID-19 cases in Korea is ongoing. The government increased Seoul's social distancing to the 2.5 level, and the number of confirmed cases is increasing daily. Due to a shortage of hospital beds, treatment is difficult. Furthermore, gatherings at the end of the year and the beginning of next year are expected to worsen the effects. The purpose of this paper is to emphasize the importance of prediction timing rather than prediction of the number of confirmed cases. Thus, in this study, five groups were set according to minimum, maximum, and high variability. Through empirical data analysis, the groups were subdivided into a total of 19 cases. The cumulative number of COVID-19 confirmed cases is predicted using the auto regressive integrated moving average (ARIMA) model and compared with the actual number of confirmed cases. Through group and case-by-case prediction, forecasts can accurately determine decreasing and increasing trends. To prevent further spread of COVID-19, urgent and strong government restrictions are needed. This study will help the government and the Korea Disease Control and Prevention Agency (KDCA) to respond systematically to a future surge in confirmed cases.

Keywords: time-series; ARIMA; forecasting; confirmed cases; COVID-19; pandemic

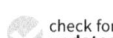

Citation: Lee, D.H.; Kim, Y.S.; Koh, Y.Y.; Song, K.Y.; Chang, I.H. Forecasting COVID-19 Confirmed Cases Using Empirical Data Analysis in Korea. *Healthcare* **2021**, *9*, 254. https://doi.org/10.3390/healthcare9030254

Academic Editor: Manoj Sharma

Received: 31 December 2020
Accepted: 19 February 2021
Published: 1 March 2021

Publisher's Note: MDPI stays neutral with regard to jurisdictional claims in published maps and institutional affiliations.

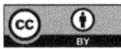

Copyright: © 2021 by the authors. Licensee MDPI, Basel, Switzerland. This article is an open access article distributed under the terms and conditions of the Creative Commons Attribution (CC BY) license (https://creativecommons.org/licenses/by/4.0/).

1. Introduction

The COVID-19 pandemic has had a significant impact on human life. The G20 Summit held in a virtual conference on March 2020 to discuss pending global issues resulting from COVID-19. Coping and confronting the pandemic includes activities such as protecting lives, protecting jobs and income, restoring trust, preserving financial stability, restoring growth, minimizing disruption of trade and global supply chains, and providing assistance to countries in need of support. COVID-19 has caused major economic losses, paralyzing national economies around the world. The International Monetary Fund (IMF) predicted that global trade volume would shrink by 10.4% on-year [1]. The World Bank Group (WBG) is expecting that the global trade volume will drop 5.2% and to have its worst year since World War II [2].

COVID-19 has been called a novel coronavirus (2019-nCoV), but on 11 March 2020, the World Health Organization (WHO) announced its official name as COVID-19 [3]. On 13 February 2020, the International Committee on Taxonomy of Viruses (ICTV) officially announced the virus' name as SARS-CoV-2. Coronavirus is a ribonucleic acid (RNA) virus that causes respiratory diseases, such as colds. It was named coronavirus because its outer skin is shaped like a crown surrounded by bumps. It causes infection in a variety of animals, including humans. The WHO classifies pandemic alarm levels from 1 to 6, according to the infectious disease risk. This pandemic corresponds to the highest warning level—6. When an infectious disease spreads worldwide and spreads across continents, it is called a pandemic. Thus far, the WHO has declared three pandemics: the Hong Kong Flu in 1968, the Swine Flu in 2009, and COVID-19 in 2020 [4].

Until recently, the top five affected countries were as follows: the United States death toll record with 17 million, India with 10 million, Brazil with 7 million, Russia with 2.7 million, and France with 2.4 million. In terms of death rate, Mexico has the highest death rate at 9.1%, China has 5.3%, Iran has 4.7%, and Italy has 3.5%. In Korea, the cumulative number of confirmed cases is about 47,000, and the death rate is approximately 1.4% [5].

Various studies have been conducted on past pandemic infections and disease. Guan et al. [6] predicted the incidence of hepatitis A virus (HAV) using an auto regressive integrated moving average (ARIMA) model and an artificial neural network (ANN). Earnest et al. [7] forecasted the number of confirmed cases by applying the ARIMA model to the number of confirmed cases per day for severe acute respiratory syndrome (SARS). By applying ARIMA to China's HFRS data, Liu et al. [8] predicted the incidence of hemorrhagic fever with renal syndrome (HFRS) from 2009 to 2011. Wu et al. [9] predicted the incidence of HFRS over one year by using a hybrid model that combines ARIMA, a generalized regression neural network (GRNN), and the non-linear autoregressive neural network (NARNN) with ARIMA. Nsoesie et al. [10] tried to predict the hantavirus pulmonary syndrome (HPS) using an ARIMA model. Chen et al. [11] used the seasonal autoregressive integrated moving average (SARIMA) to predict the incidence of influenza in China; they found that the incidence rate varies according to region and season.

Based on past infectious diseases, research related to COVID-19 has also been actively conducted. Using a differential equation model that reflected social distancing and transmission rate as parameters, Webb et al. [12] predicted and compared the number of confirmed cases considering the number of report and the presence of symptoms in Italy, Spain, and Korea. This demonstrates the importance of controlling COVID-19 infection through social distancing. Alakus et al. [13] developed a prediction algorithm using deep learning and had a positive impact on clinical prediction studies of COVID-19. Pham [14] studied the cumulative number of deaths, the mortality per capita per unit time, and the maximum total number of deaths as functions, and the solution of differential equations composed of the functions is proposed as the numerical model of COVID-19. Pham [15] generalized by introducing a function of recovered cases to the model in [14]. Additionally, Pham [16] developed a new mathematical model by introducing the time-dependent effort of social restrictions—the resumption of states, wearing masks, and social distancing. Arias et al. [17] suggested a generalized logistics regression to predict the number of cases of COVID-19.

In addition to the aforementioned methods, studies have also been conducted using the ARIMA model to estimate the spread of COVID-19, examples of which are as follows. Using ARIMA and Richard's model, Kumar et al. [18] conducted a study that forecast the population impact of COVID-19 in India compare goodness-of-fit for models. Petropoulos et al. [19] predicted the number of COVID-19 patients in a short period of time using a simple time series in Denmark, Norway, and Sweden. Additionally, [19] tracked and compared the stringency level of each country. Using the ARIMA model, Ceylan [20] predicted the number of COVID-19 cases in Italy, Spain, and France. Alzahrani et al. [21] forecasted the number of COVID-19 confirmed cases in Saudi Arabia for the next four weeks. Yang et al. [22] predicted the number of cases in Italy for the next few days. Kufel [23] presented ARIMA to forecast the rate of infection in 32 European countries over the next seven days. In addition, there is a variety of research that studies the impact of COVID-19 [24–30].

In this paper, we apply the ARIMA model and empirical data analysis to forecast the number of confirmed COVID-19 cases in Korea. Using actual data, dividing the wave into several cases, predicting the number of cumulative confirmed cases for each case, and comparing the criteria. In doing so, we emphasize the importance of timing of forecasting to make a meaningful forecast. In particular, the period from 20 January 2020 (first confirmed case) to 26 October 2020 (the beginning of the third wave of COVID-19) is divided into five groups, which are subdivided into a total of 19 cases (the division is detailed in Section 2). Section 2 briefly describes the material and methods. Additionally, the current status of confirmed cases in Korea, empirical data analysis of group and case information, ARIMA models, and criteria are introduced. Section 3 presents the analysis and results. Section 4 concludes the paper.

2. Material and Methods

2.1. The Number of COVID-19 Confirmed Cases in Korea

Figure 1 shows the number of confirmed cases and cumulative confirmed cases by month in Korea [31]. On 20 January 2020, a tourist from Wuhan became the first confirmed case in Korea. Then, 11 cases were reported, bringing the cumulative number of confirmed cases to 12. In February and March, the number of confirmed cases increased sharply. The primary cause of infections was indoor religious gatherings. Within three months of the first outbreak, the cumulative number of confirmed cases reached 9887. The period between February and April 2020 is defined as the first wave of COVID-19 in Korea [31,32].

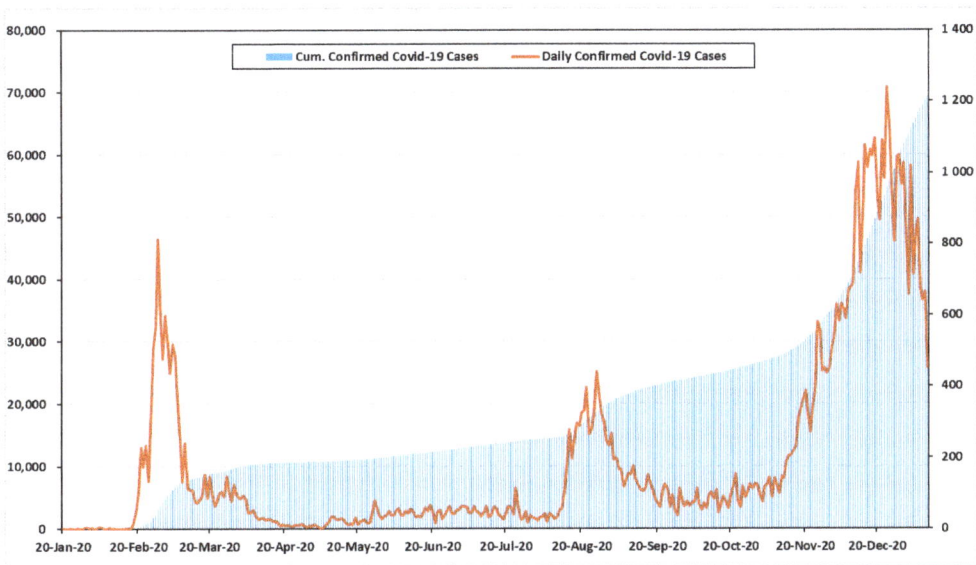

Figure 1. The number of confirmed cases and cumulative confirmed cases of COVID-19 in Korea in 2020 (including imported cases).

After the first wave, the number of confirmed cases decreased rapidly and there was a stable infection rate across the country. Nevertheless, in August and September, the second wave was generated by political rallies and church gatherings. During the second wave, the cases increased sharply, and the government raised social distancing to level 2. There were 2757 cases in October, which was only slightly lower than in September. This period showed a stable infection rate, in comparison to other waves, but it included the day with the largest increase in confirmed cases; this study did not thoroughly address the third wave, because it is still underway [31,33].

From November to present, the number of confirmed cases increased rapidly again. This is defined as the third wave. In November, the total number of cases was 8017. Small gatherings among families and friends accounted for more than 20% of the third wave's infections. Some of the provincial governments decided to raise the social distancing level to 2.5, which is the second highest. Worst of all, the confirmed cases in Seoul are being housed in retrofitted containers because of hospital bed shortages. The government and citizens fear the need to raise social distancing to level 3 [31,34].

All information related to confirmed cases in this paper was provided by the government and was aggregated daily at midnight (00:00) [31].

2.2. Information of Groups and Cases Using Empirical Data Analysis

2.2.1. Empirical Data Analysis

Empirical analysis is an evidence-based approach to the study and interpretation of information. The empirical approach relies on real-world data, metrics, and results, rather than theories and concepts. Empirical analysis is a common approach used to study probable answers through quantified observations of empirical evidence. However, empirical analysis never gives an absolute answer, only the most likely answer based on probability.

We can formulate the increasing number of confirmed cases of COVID-19 as follows:

$$y'(t) = \lim_{\Delta t \to 0} \frac{y(t + \Delta t) - y(t)}{\Delta t} \quad (1)$$

where $y'(t)$ illustrates the increasing number of confirmed cases of COVID-19 during the time interval Δt. Then, $y(t)$ is the observed cumulative number of confirmed cases of COVID-19 over time t. Therefore, $y(t + \Delta t)$ denotes the observed cumulative number of confirmed cases of COVID-19 over time $t + \Delta t$. Given different values of Δt, we are interested in investigating the pattern of $y'(t)$.

2.2.2. Information of Groups and Cases

Figure 2 shows the increasing number of confirmed cases of COVID-19 during the time interval Δt. As shown in Figure 2, the five points of high variability were divided and examined in detail. The criteria for defining the five groups are as follows: Group 1 and Group 4 were based on the day when the number of confirmed cases per day was the highest in the first and second waves. Group 2 was based on the day when the number of confirmed cases was the lowest. Last, Group 3 and Group 5 were based on the days with the greatest variability (the point at which more than 100 confirmed cases began to appear), which signaled the beginning of the second and third waves.

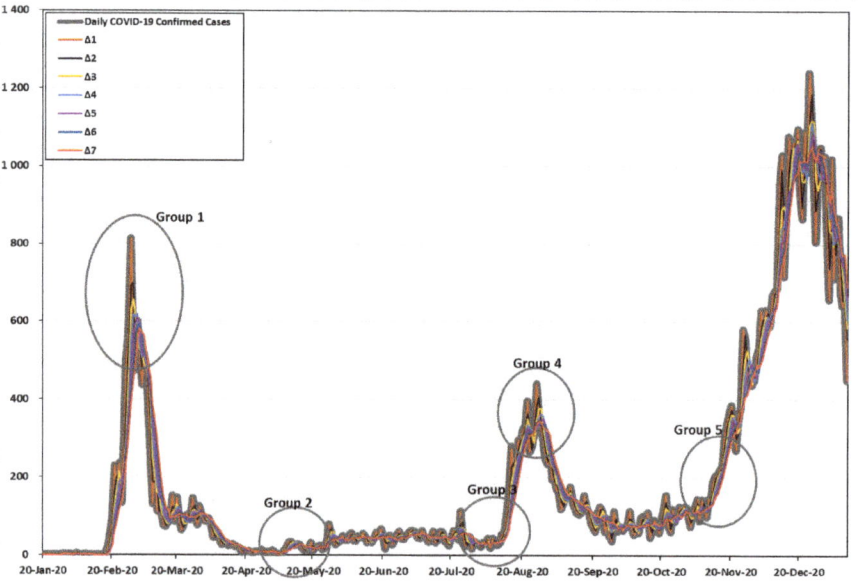

Figure 2. The increasing number of confirmed cases of COVID-19 by time interval.

Details can be found in Table 1. In Group 1, with the time interval $\Delta t = 1$, the maximum frequency was 813 cases (28 February 2020), the time intervals $\Delta t = 2$–4 were 699.5, 656.7, and 618.8 cases (29 February 2020), and the time internals $\Delta t = 4$–5 were 618.8 and 609.2 cases (2 March 2020). Time internals $\Delta t = 6$–7 were 593.7 and 581.0 cases (3 March 2020) in the first wave of the COVID-19 pandemic, respectively.

Table 1. The number of confirmed cases of COVID-19 during time interval Δt by Group.

Group	Date	Number of Confirmed Cases of COVID-19		Number of Confirmed Cases of COVID-19 during Time Interval Δt						
		Daily	Cum.	$\Delta t=1$	$\Delta t=2$	$\Delta t=3$	$\Delta t=4$	$\Delta t=5$	$\Delta t=6$	$\Delta t=7$
Group 1	27 February 2020	571	2337	571.0	538.0	453.3	373.5	345.8	317.3	304.7
	28 February 2020	813	3150	813.0	692.0	629.7	543.3	461.4	423.7	388.1
	29 February 2020	586	3736	586.0	699.5	656.7	618.8	551.8	482.2	446.9
	1 March 2020	476	4212	476.0	531.0	625.0	611.5	590.2	539.2	481.3
	2 March 2020	600	4812	600.0	538.0	554.0	618.8	609.2	591.8	547.9
	3 March 2020	516	5328	516.0	558.0	530.7	544.5	598.2	593.7	581.0
	4 March 2020	438	5766	438.0	477.0	518.0	507.5	523.2	571.5	571.4
Group 2	4 May 2020	3	10,804	3.0	5.5	8.0	7.5	7.8	7.2	7.4
	5 May 2020	2	10,806	2.0	2.5	4.3	6.5	6.4	6.8	6.4
	6 May 2020	4	10,810	4.0	3.0	3.0	4.3	6.0	6.0	6.4
	7 May 2020	12	10,822	12.0	8.0	6.0	5.3	5.8	7.0	6.9
	8 May 2020	18	10,840	18.0	15.0	11.3	9.0	7.8	7.8	8.6
Group 3	12 August 2020	56	14,770	56.0	55.0	48.0	43.0	41.6	41.8	38.7
	13 August 2020	103	14,873	103.0	79.5	71.0	61.8	55.0	51.8	50.6
	14 August 2020	166	15,039	166.0	134.5	108.3	94.8	82.6	73.5	68.1
	15 August 2020	279	15,318	279.0	222.5	182.7	151.0	131.6	115.3	102.9
	16 August 2020	197	15,515	197.0	238.0	214.0	186.3	160.2	142.5	127.0
Group 4	16 August 2020	320	18,265	320.0	300.0	288.7	315.8	319.0	319.8	315.3
	25 August 2020	441	18,706	441.0	380.5	347.0	326.8	340.8	339.3	337.1
	26 August 2020	371	19,077	371.0	406.0	377.3	353.0	335.6	345.8	343.9
	27 August 2020	323	19,400	323.0	347.0	378.3	363.8	347.0	333.5	342.6
	28 August 2020	299	19,699	299.0	311.0	331.0	358.5	350.8	339.0	328.6
	29 August 2020	248	19,947	248.0	273.5	290.0	310.3	336.4	333.7	326.0
Group 5	20 October 2020	91	25,424	91.0	74.5	75.0	79.0	77.8	72.7	78.0
	21 October 2020	119	25,543	119.0	105.0	89.3	86.0	87.0	84.7	79.3
	22 October 2020	155	25,698	155.0	137.0	121.7	105.8	99.8	98.3	94.7
	23 October 2020	77	25,775	77.0	116.0	117.0	110.5	100.0	96.0	95.3
	24 October 2020	61	25,836	61.0	69.0	97.7	103.0	100.6	93.5	91.0
	25 October 2020	119	25,955	119.0	90.0	85.7	103.0	106.2	103.7	97.1
	26 October 2020	88	26,043	88.0	103.5	89.3	86.3	100.0	103.2	101.4
	27 October 2020	103	26,146	103.0	95.5	103.3	92.8	89.6	100.5	103.1

In Group 2, with the time interval $\Delta t = 1$, 2, and 7, the minimum frequencies were 2, 2.5, and 6.4 cases (5 May 2020). The time intervals $\Delta t = 3$–4 and 6–7 were 3, 4.3, 6, and 6.4 cases (6 May 2020), and the time intervals $\Delta t = 5$ was 5.8 cases (7 May 2020), respectively.

In Group 3, with the time interval $\Delta t = 1$, the frequency with high variability (based on more than 100 cases) was 103 cases (13 August 2020). The time intervals $\Delta t = 2$–3 were 134.5 and 108.3 cases (14 August 2020). The time internals $\Delta t = 4$–7 were 151,

131.6, 115.3, and 102.9 cases (15 August 2020) before the second wave of the COVID-19 pandemic, respectively.

In Group 4, with the time interval $\Delta t = 1$, the maximum frequency was 441 cases (26 August 2020). The time intervals $\Delta t = 2$ and 6–7 were 406, 345.8, and 343.9 cases (27 August 2020). The time internals $\Delta t = 3$–4 were 378.3 and 363.8 cases (28 August 2020). Time internals $\Delta t = 5$ was 350.8 cases (29 August 2020) in the second wave of the COVID-19 pandemic.

In Group 5, with the time interval $\Delta t = 1$–2, the frequency with high variability (based on more than 100 cases) was 119 and 105 cases (21 October 2020). The time intervals $\Delta t = 3$–4 were 121.7 and 105.8 cases (22 October 2020). The time internals $\Delta t = 5$ was 100 cases (23 October 2020); the time internals $\Delta t = 6$ was 103.7 cases (25 October 2020); and the time internals $\Delta t = 7$ was 101.4 cases (26 October 2020) before the third wave of the COVID-19 pandemic, respectively.

As shown in Table 2, we set cases by date for forecast analysis based on the time point mentioned in each group. In addition, it was used for predictive analysis using the data up to the mentioned time point.

Table 2. Groups and cases by period for forecast analysis.

Group	Case	Date	Group	Case	Date
1	Case 1	20 January 2020~28 February 2020	4	Case 11	20 January 2020~26 August 2020
	Case 2	20 January 2020~29 February 2020		Case 12	20 January 2020~27 August 2020
	Case 3	20 January 2020~2 March 2020		Case 13	20 January 2020~28 August 2020
	Case 4	20 January 2020~2 March 2020		Case 14	20 January 2020~29 August 2020
2	Case 5	20 January 2020~5 May 2020	5	Case 15	20 January 2020~21 October 2020
	Case 6	20 January 2020~6 May 2020		Case 16	20 January 2020~22 October 2020
	Case 7	20 January 2020~7 May 2020		Case 17	20 January 2020~23 October 2020
3	Case 8	20 January 2020~13 August 2020		Case 18	20 January 2020~25 October 2020
	Case 9	20 January 2020~14 August 2020		Case 19	20 January 2020~26 October 2020
	Case 10	20 January 2020~15 August 2020	Recent Case		20 January 2020~27 October 2020

2.3. Time Series

In the autoregressive (AR) model, the partial autocorrelation coefficient (PAC) had a significant spike, and the autocorrelation coefficient (AC) decreased in sequence. In this case, the order of AR (p) is determined based on the number of significant spikes of the PAC. The formula for the AR (p) model is as follows:

$$Y_t = \epsilon_t + \alpha_1 Y_{t-1} + \alpha_2 Y_{t-2} + \cdots \alpha_p Y_{t-p} \qquad (2)$$

Unlike AR, in the moving average (MA) model, the AC has a significant spike. The PAC decreases in sequence, and the order q of the MA model is determined based on the number of significant spikes of the AC. The formula for the MA (q) model is as follows:

$$Y_t = \epsilon_t - \beta_1 \epsilon_{t-1} - \beta_2 \epsilon_{t-2} - \cdots \beta_q \epsilon_{t-q} \tag{3}$$

The autoregressive moving average (ARMA) model shows a form of sequentially decreasing in both the AC and the PAC. The formula is as follows:

$$Y_t = \alpha_1 Y_{t-1} + \alpha_2 Y_{t-2} + \cdots \alpha_p Y_{t-p} + \epsilon_t - \beta_1 \epsilon_{t-1} - \beta_2 \epsilon_{t-2} - \cdots \beta_q \epsilon_{t-q} \tag{4}$$

where ϵ_t is called the error or white noise. The ϵ_t is assumed to be independently normal distribution. The ARIMA model converts a non-stationary time series data into a stationary time series that is expressed as ARIMA (p,d,q), where p is the order of the AR model, d is the differencing order, and q is the order of the MA model. For example, AR (1) is equivalent to ARIMA (1,0,0), and MA (2) is equivalent to ARIMA (0,0,2).

There is no clear trend in the stationary time series, and the average and variance are constant over time. In the case of a known time series analysis model, analysis is possible when the data is in the form of time series data that shows normality without trend or seasonality. In the case of data having a long period, a trend with a sudden and unpredictable change in direction, or data showing seasonality, the analysis is conducted after making the data in the form of a stationary time series through the difference using the difference between observed values. To check whether it is a normal time series or a non-stationary time series, check through a sequence chart or ACF (auto correlation function) [35].

This paper dealt only with the ARIMA (p,2,q) model. In general, a non-stationary time series becomes a stationary time series by a first or second differencing. In the data of this study, when the difference was 0 or 1, the sequence chart had an inconsistent form of mean and variance, and it can be seen that the ACF had an abnormal time series in the form of slowly decreasing. When the difference was 2, the mean and variance appeared in a certain form, indicating that the time series was normal.

When d = 1, the cumulative number of confirmed cases predicted by the ARIMA model, gradually decreased or showed a negative value, which is a contradiction. However, when d = 2, the predicted value of the cumulative cases increased stably, so the ARIMA (p,2,q) model was used.

2.4. Criteria for the Comparion of Goodness-of-Fit

To compare the goodness-of-fit by ARIMA for each case, the following four criteria were used:

First, root mean square error (RMSE) is as follows:

$$\text{RMSE} = \sqrt{\frac{1}{n} \sum_{t=1}^{n} e_t^2} \tag{5}$$

Second, mean absolute error (MAE) is as follows:

$$\text{MAE} = \frac{1}{n} \sum_{t=1}^{n} |e_t^2| \tag{6}$$

Third, mean absolute percentage error (MAPE) is as follows:

$$\text{MAPE} = \frac{100}{n} \sum_{t=1}^{n} e_t^2 \tag{7}$$

Finally, the sum of square error (SSE) is as follows:

$$\text{SSE} = \sum_{t=n+1}^{(n+1)+14} (Y_t - \hat{Y}_t)^2 \qquad (8)$$

Here, e_t is the difference (error) between the actual cumulative number of cases Y_t and the predicted value $\hat{Y}_t$ of the ARIMA model at time t. Additionally, n is the length of time t. The SSE was calculated as the difference between the predicted values and the data for 14 days—two weeks from the end of the truncated case. The smaller the values of all four criteria mentioned above, the better the fit, relative to other models.

3. Results

For the data set, the time series method was applied to compare the criteria of each section using SPSS 25 (IBM, Armonk, NY, USA). The ARIMA (p,d,q) models were fitted p = 0, 1, ... , 5, d = 2, q = 0, 1, ... , 5 for 19 cases, with 684 models to be compared. Among them, only the top six models of each case were selected based on the RMSE.

3.1. Prediction of Cumulative Confirmed Cases of COVID-19 by Group and Case Using ARIMA
3.1.1. Comparison of Goodness-of-Fit by Group and Case

Tables 3–7 show the fitting ARIMA models and criteria for groups and cases, and sorts by RMSE (in ascending order).

Table 3. Results of auto regressive integrated moving average (ARIMA) models for Group 1 (Case 1–4).

Case	Model	RMSE	MAPE	MAE
1	ARIMA (5,2,5)	41.181	279.699	21.819
	ARIMA (5,2,3)	43.399	248.562	24.118
	ARIMA (5,2,4)	43.842	245.299	23.871
	ARIMA (5,2,2)	43.898	210.373	23.854
	ARIMA (3,2,3)	44.380	170.642	22.634
	ARIMA (4,2,2)	44.985	186.538	25.879
2	ARIMA (5,2,5)	41.618	280.246	22.416
	ARIMA (5,2,4)	42.445	264.567	23.586
	ARIMA (4,2,5)	43.134	185.019	23.488
	ARIMA (5,2,3)	43.212	233.869	24.876
	ARIMA (4,2,4)	43.358	197.110	25.585
	ARIMA (4,2,2)	44.134	180.253	25.783
3	ARIMA (5,2,5)	49.641	162.569	25.548
	ARIMA (5,2,4)	53.291	185.799	28.713
	ARIMA (5,2,3)	53.474	185.343	29.178
	ARIMA (4,2,3)	53.571	197.765	31.706
	ARIMA (4,2,4)	54.185	196.412	31.613
	ARIMA (5,2,1)	56.478	200.521	33.533
4	ARIMA (5,2,5)	49.869	149.950	25.762
	ARIMA (5,2,2)	52.173	177.074	29.535
	ARIMA (5,2,4)	52.491	172.811	28.209
	ARIMA (5,2,3)	52.593	177.511	28.595
	ARIMA (4,2,4)	53.320	191.480	30.849
	ARIMA (4,2,3)	53.340	184.271	30.593

Table 4. Results of ARIMA models for Group 2 (case 5–7).

Case	Model	RMSE	MAPE	MAE
5	ARIMA (2,2,5)	56.172	5.963	27.920
	ARIMA (5,2,5)	56.428	5.968	27.800
	ARIMA (3,2,5)	56.471	5.885	28.122
	ARIMA (4,2,5)	56.711	5.965	28.064
	ARIMA (5,2,3)	56.901	5.805	28.879
	ARIMA (1,2,5)	57.573	5.741	29.995
6	ARIMA (2,2,5)	55.895	5.719	27.720
	ARIMA (5,2,5)	56.147	5.748	27.637
	ARIMA (3,2,5)	56.185	5.668	27.886
	ARIMA (4,2,5)	56.424	5.708	27.934
	ARIMA (5,2,3)	56.589	5.737	28.651
	ARIMA (1,2,5)	57.283	5.719	29.760
7	ARIMA (2,2,5)	55.629	5.656	27.576
	ARIMA (5,2,5)	55.856	5.705	27.451
	ARIMA (3,2,5)	55.911	5.697	27.726
	ARIMA (4,2,5)	56.074	5.880	27.739
	ARIMA (5,2,3)	56.314	5.772	28.552
	ARIMA (1,2,5)	57.000	5.821	29.559

Table 5. Results of ARIMA models for Group 3 (case 8–10).

Case	Model	RMSE	MAPE	MAE
8	ARIMA (2,2,5)	41.712	3.338	21.422
	ARIMA (3,2,5)	41.842	3.324	21.452
	ARIMA (5,2,4)	41.908	3.357	21.539
	ARIMA (5,2,3)	42.149	3.332	21.863
	ARIMA (1,2,5)	42.659	3.443	22.016
	ARIMA (4,2,5)	43.019	3.400	21.602
9	ARIMA (2,2,5)	41.912	3.826	21.639
	ARIMA (3,2,5)	41.948	3.929	21.489
	ARIMA (5,2,3)	42.327	3.750	21.909
	ARIMA (5,2,4)	42.670	3.789	22.007
	ARIMA (1,2,5)	42.830	3.941	22.299
	ARIMA (4,2,5)	43.182	3.658	21.863
10	ARIMA (2,2,5)	42.796	5.012	22.084
	ARIMA (4,2,5)	42.953	4.557	22.098
	ARIMA (5,2,4)	42.961	4.570	22.007
	ARIMA (5,2,3)	43.140	5.146	22.399
	ARIMA (1,2,5)	43.640	5.178	22.863
	ARIMA (2,2,3)	44.011	4.337	22.637

Table 6. Results of ARIMA models for Group 4 (case 11–14).

Case	Model	RMSE	MAPE	MAE
11	ARIMA (5,2,5)	44.253	5.333	23.426
	ARIMA (3,2,5)	44.313	5.304	23.198
	ARIMA (4,2,5)	44.417	5.334	23.291
	ARIMA (2,2,5)	44.558	5.417	23.484
	ARIMA (5,2,3)	44.904	5.330	23.665
	ARIMA (5,2,4)	45.051	5.390	23.746
12	ARIMA (3,2,5)	44.405	4.711	23.263
	ARIMA (4,2,5)	44.476	4.797	23.207
	ARIMA (2,2,5)	44.643	4.866	23.504
	ARIMA (5,2,3)	45.015	4.755	23.653
	ARIMA (5,2,4)	45.314	4.626	23.801
	ARIMA (1,2,5)	45.397	4.467	23.848
13	ARIMA (3,2,5)	44.471	4.190	23.417
	ARIMA (4,2,5)	44.536	4.313	23.344
	ARIMA (2,2,5)	44.675	4.372	23.506
	ARIMA (5,2,4)	44.779	4.452	23.463
	ARIMA (5,2,5)	44.798	4.352	23.527
	ARIMA (4,2,4)	44.867	4.352	23.050
14	ARIMA (3,2,5)	44.449	3.845	23.491
	ARIMA (4,2,5)	44.484	4.056	23.391
	ARIMA (5,2,4)	44.707	4.247	23.410
	ARIMA (5,2,5)	44.714	4.188	23.457
	ARIMA (4,2,4)	44.773	4.242	22.997
	ARIMA (5,2,3)	44.941	4.116	23.740

Table 7. Results of ARIMA models for Group 5 (case 15–19).

Case	Model	RMSE	MAPE	MAE
15	ARIMA (3,2,5)	41.744	2.511	23.107
	ARIMA (4,2,5)	41.811	2.513	23.150
	ARIMA (2,2,5)	41.892	2.495	23.300
	ARIMA (5,2,3)	42.234	2.524	23.307
	ARIMA (5,2,4)	42.308	2.536	23.433
	ARIMA (1,2,5)	42.622	2.509	23.948
16	ARIMA (4,2,5)	41.852	2.647	23.268
	ARIMA (2,2,5)	41.932	2.624	23.408
	ARIMA (5,2,3)	42.285	2.636	23.714
	ARIMA (5,2,4)	42.319	2.651	23.534
	ARIMA (1,2,5)	42.631	2.628	24.053
	ARIMA (4,2,4)	42.779	2.609	23.730

Table 7. Cont.

Case	Model	RMSE	MAPE	MAE
17	ARIMA (3,2,5)	41.957	2.429	23.375
	ARIMA (4,2,5)	42.030	2.428	23.410
	ARIMA (2,2,5)	42.100	2.419	23.532
	ARIMA (5,2,3)	42.416	2.432	23.727
	ARIMA (1,2,5)	42.782	2.414	24.175
	ARIMA (4,2,4)	42.892	2.458	23.869
18	ARIMA (3,2,5)	41.938	2.444	23.457
	ARIMA (2,2,5)	42.072	2.449	23.619
	ARIMA (5,2,4)	42.349	2.489	23.824
	ARIMA (5,2,3)	42.366	2.472	23.791
	ARIMA (5,2,5)	42.390	2.498	23.826
	ARIMA (1,2,5)	42.714	2.447	24.212
19	ARIMA (3,2,5)	41.871	2.392	23.431
	ARIMA (4,2,5)	41.940	2.391	23.491
	ARIMA (2,2,5)	42.005	2.397	23.589
	ARIMA (5,2,2)	42.278	2.386	23.846
	ARIMA (5,2,3)	42.319	2.398	23.796
	ARIMA (5,2,5)	42.401	2.394	23.943

As can be seen in Table 3, in case 1, the RMSE of ARIMA (5,2,5) was 41.181, which was closer to the actual data than other models. In addition, the MAE of the model was 21.819, which was the smallest of all models. The MAPE of ARIMA (3,2,3) was 170.642, which was the smallest among case 1. In case 2, the RMSE and MAE of ARIMA (5,2,5) were the smallest. Based on MAPE, the value of ARIMA (4,2,2) was the closest to the actual data. In Cases 3 and 4, all criteria of ARIMA (5,2,5) appeared to be predictive models with the best descriptive.

As can be seen in Table 4, in case 5, the RMSE of ARIMA (2,2,5) was 56.172, which was the smallest among case 5. Based on MAPE, the value of ARIMA (1,2,5) was 5.741, which was the smallest. The MAE of ARIMA (5,2,5) was 27.800, which was the smallest. In case 6, based on the RMSE, the value of ARIMA (2,2,5) was 55.895, which was the smallest. The MAPE of ARIMA (3,2,5) was 5.668, which appeared to be a predictive model with the best descriptive. The MAE of ARIMA (5,2,5) was 27.637, which was the smallest. In case 7, the RMSE and MAPE of ARIMA (2,2,5) were the closest among case 7, and the MAE of ARIMA (5,2,5) was the smallest of all the models.

As can be seen in Table 5, in case 8, the RMSE and MAE of ARIMA (2,2,5) were the closest among case 8. The MAPE of ARIMA (3,2,5) was 3.324, which was the smallest among the other models. In case 9, the RMSE of ARIMA (2,2,5), the MAPE of ARIMA (4,2,5), and the MAE of ARIMA (3,2,5) were 41.912, 3.658, and 21.489, which were the closest to the actual data in comparison to the other models. In case 10, the RMSE of ARIMA (2,2,5) was 42.796, which was the closest to the others. The MAPE of ARIMA (2,2,3) and the MAE of ARIMA (5,2,4) appeared to be predictive models with the best goodness-of-fit.

As can be seen in Table 6, in case 11, the RMSE of ARIMA (5,2,5) was 44.253, which was closer to the actual data than the other models. Based on the MAPE and MAE, the values of ARIMA (3,2,5) were the closest among case 11. In case 12, the RMSE of ARIMA (3,2,5) was 44.405, which appeared to be the best predictive value. The MAPE of ARIMA (1,2,5) was 4.467, which was the smallest. The MAE of ARIMA (4,2,5) was 23.207, which was the closest to the others. In cases 13 and 14, the RMSE and MAPE of ARIMA (3,2,5) provided the best fit. Based on MAE, ARIMA (4,2,4) appeared to be a predictive model with the best fit.

As can be seen in Table 7, in case 15, the RMSE and MAE of ARIMA (3,2,5) provided the best fit. The MAPE of ARIMA (2,2,5) was 2.495, which was closer to the actual data than the other models. In case 16, the RMSE and MAE of ARIMA (4,2,5) provided the best fit. The MAPE of ARIMA (4,2,4) was 2.609, which predicted significantly better results than the others. In case 17, as in case 15, the RMSE and MAE of ARIMA (3,2,5) show the best fit. The MAPE of ARIMA (1,2,5) was the smallest. In case 18, all criteria of ARIMA (3,2,5) provided the best fit among the other models. In case 19, as in case 15, the RMSE and MAE of ARIMA (3,2,5) were predictive with the best fit. The MAPE of ARIMA (5,2,2) was 2.386, which was the closest to the actual data.

3.1.2. Comparison of Predictive Value by Group and Case

Table 8 describes the results of the ARIMA models for each group and case, based on SSE. Here, note means the time interval, including the variability (maximum, minimum, and high variability of the point at which more than 100 confirmed cases began to appear), elapsed from the base date of each group.

Table 8. Results of ARIMA models for each group and case based on SSE.

Group	Case	Model	SSE	Rank of SSE	Note
1	2	ARIMA (4,2,5)	138,245,907	1	$\Delta t = 2, 3, 4$
	4	ARIMA (5,2,5)	159,104,779	2	$\Delta t = 6, 7$
	3	ARIMA (5,2,5)	195,270,591	3	$\Delta t = 4, 5$
	3	ARIMA (5,2,4)	273,033,961	4	$\Delta t = 4, 5$
	4	ARIMA (5,2,4)	311,756,668	5	$\Delta t = 6, 7$
2	7	ARIMA (5,2,5)	21,750	1	$\Delta t = 5$
	5	ARIMA (5,2,5)	978,159	2	$\Delta t = 1, 2, 7$
	6	ARIMA (5,2,5)	182,580,231	3	$\Delta t = 3, 4, 6, 7$
	6	ARIMA (1,2,5)	250,929,996	4	$\Delta t = 3, 4, 6, 7$
	5	ARIMA (4,2,5)	282,621,031	5	$\Delta t = 1, 2, 7$
3	10	ARIMA (1,2,5)	16,973,894	1	$\Delta t = 4, 5, 6, 7$
	9	ARIMA (4,2,5)	28,752,738	2	$\Delta t = 2, 3$
	9	ARIMA (5,2,3)	311,216,609	3	$\Delta t = 2, 3$
	8	ARIMA (5,2,3)	360,558,068	4	$\Delta t = 1$
	8	ARIMA (5,2,4)	948,734,643	5	$\Delta t = 1$
4	14	ARIMA (4,2,5)	26,281,173	1	$\Delta t = 5$
	14	ARIMA (5,2,3)	30,701,687	2	$\Delta t = 5$
	12	ARIMA (5,2,3)	39,839,429	3	$\Delta t = 2, 6, 7$
	12	ARIMA (4,2,5)	43,645,283	4	$\Delta t = 2, 6, 7$
	11	ARIMA (5,2,3)	47,148,618	5	$\Delta t = 1$
5	17	ARIMA (2,2,5)	45,812	1	$\Delta t = 5$
	18	ARIMA (3,2,5)	48,181	2	$\Delta t = 6$
	19	ARIMA (3,2,5)	64,905	3	$\Delta t = 7$
	15	ARIMA (1,2,5)	397,393	4	$\Delta t = 1, 2$
	19	ARIMA (2,2,5)	2,161,447	5	$\Delta t = 7$

As can be seen in Table 8, in Group 1, the SSE of ARIMA (4,2,5) for case 2 was 138,245,907, which was significantly smaller than the others. In Group 2, the SSE of ARIMA (5,2,5) for case 7 was 21,750, which was the smallest. The SSE of ARIMA (1,2,5) for case 10 in Group 3, ARIMA (4,2,5) for case 14 in Group 4, and ARIMA (2,2,5) for case 17 in Group 5 were the closest to actual data compared to the other models in the same group. We confirmed that the analysis should be performed taking into account the time interval of the last five days or more, including the maximum, minimum, and high variability (when more than 100 confirmed cases started to appear).

For reference, it was confirmed that the analysis should be performed taking into account the time interval of the last five days or more, including the maximum, minimum, and high degeneration (when more than 100 confirmed cases started to appear).

Note the consideration of the maximum, minimum, and expensive modification, (a confirmed case is the time more than 100 people begin to appear) over the last five days, confirmed that this analysis should be done.

Based on the note above, Δt of the best model in Group 1 was 2, 3, and 4, a period that was the initial period of the COVID-19 outbreak. Thus, its data was small; Δt was smaller than other groups. In Groups 2, 4, and 5, the values of the best models for each group were 5. In Group 3, Δt of the best model was 4, 5, 6, and 7 and the minimum was 4. That is, we found that the best prediction in Group 3 was to analyze it using the data up to the point of high variability (minimum and maximum) over four days. Except for Group 1, which was unstable due to low data, the remaining groups were required to predict using the data up to the point of high variability (minimum and maximum) for the last five days.

3.2. Results of Fitting and Forecasting for the Latest Period Using ARIMA

The ARIMA model was fitted to the data set of confirmed COVID-19 cases, including the data set from the latest period of the third wave outbreak (up to 27 December 2020). As in Section 3.1.1, ARIMA (p,d,q) models were fitted $p = 0, 1, \ldots, 5$, $d = 2$, $q = 0, 1, \ldots, 5$ for 19 cases. Table 9 lists the top 10 based on the RMSE among the fitted ARIMA models.

Table 9. Criteria of confirmed cases according to ARIMA.

Model	RMSE	MAPE	MAE
ARIMA (3,2,5)	53.031	4.190	29.780
ARIMA (5,2,4)	53.323	4.216	29.925
ARIMA (2,2,5)	53.333	4.449	30.232
ARIMA (5,2,3)	53.591	4.120	30.061
ARIMA (4,2,3)	54.150	4.914	30.567
ARIMA (4,2,4)	54.177	4.811	30.602
ARIMA (5,2,5)	54.638	4.296	30.976
ARIMA (1,2,5)	54.680	3.860	30.569
ARIMA (3,2,4)	55.385	4.568	31.593
ARIMA (0,2,5)	55.621	4.609	30.879

Based on the RMSE, ARIMA (3,2,5) provides the best fit, the value was 53.031. Additionally, the MAE of the model was 29.780, the closest to actual model than others. Compared to other models based on MAPE, the value of ARIMA (1,2,5) was 3.860, appeared to be the best predictive model. The model with the least SSE in each group in Table 8 also had smaller RMSE, MAPE, and MAE values compared to cases in the same group. Therefore, we estimated the predicted values and 95% confidence intervals over the next 14 days for the best models, ARIMA (3,2,5) and ARIMA (1,2,5) based on three criteria.

Table 10 shows the predicted values, UCL (upper confidence limit), and LCL (lower confidence limit). According to Table 10, the number of cumulative confirmed cases for the next 14 days might be 58,532–70,389 in ARIMA (3,2,5), and 58,533–69,877 in ARIMA (1,2,5). Figures 3 and 4 show the predicted values, 95% confidence intervals, and actual data values for each model.

Table 10. Prediction of cumulative confirmed cases according to the best models with 95% confidence interval.

Date	Real Data	Based on RMSE and MAE ARIMA (3,2,5)			Based on MAPE ARIMA (1,2,5)		
		Forecast	UCL	LCL	Forecast	UCL	LCL
28 December 2020	58,714	58,532	58,636	58,427	58,533	58,640	58,425
29 December 2020	59,764	59,456	59,668	59,243	59,477	59,697	59,256
30 December 2020	60,731	60,428	60,756	60,101	60,417	60,755	60,079
31 December 2020	61,758	61,448	61,912	60,984	61,358	61,832	60,883
1 January 2021	62,578	62,432	63,046	61,818	62,248	62,875	61,622
2 January 2021	63,235	63,327	64,106	62,547	63,113	63,920	62,306
3 January 2021	64,255	64,153	65,125	63,180	63,964	64,983	62,945
4 January 2021	64,969	64,975	66,175	63,775	64,809	66,070	63,548
5 January 2021	65,807	65,847	67,308	64,386	65,651	67,181	64,121
6 January 2021	66,676	66,770	68,515	65,025	66,493	68,318	64,669
7 January 2021	67,350	67,710	69,752	65,667	67,336	69,477	65,195
8 January 2021	67,991	68,628	70,978	66,278	68,181	70,660	65,702
9 January 2021	68,648	69,515	72,185	66,845	69,028	71,864	66,192
10 January 2021	69,099	70,389	73,394	67,384	69,877	73,088	66,665

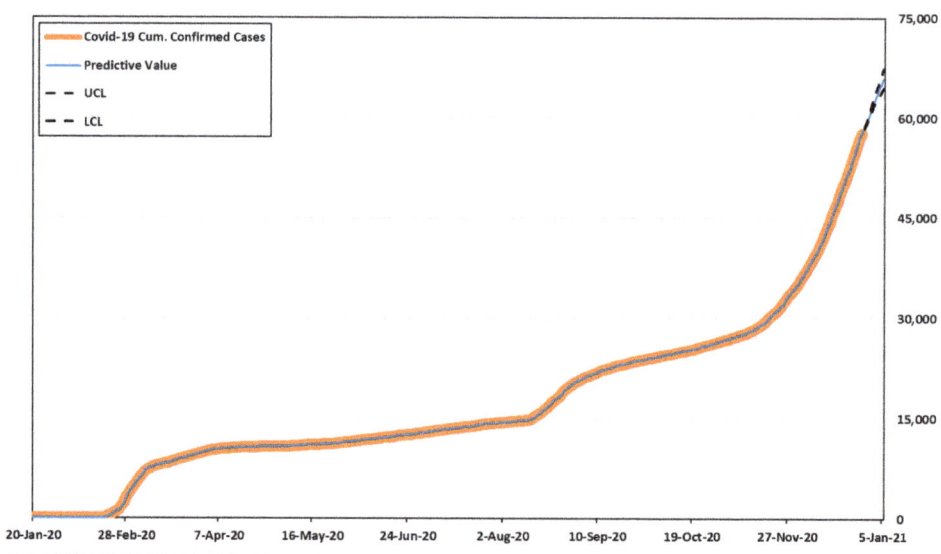

Figure 3. Time-series plot for ARIMA (3,2,5).

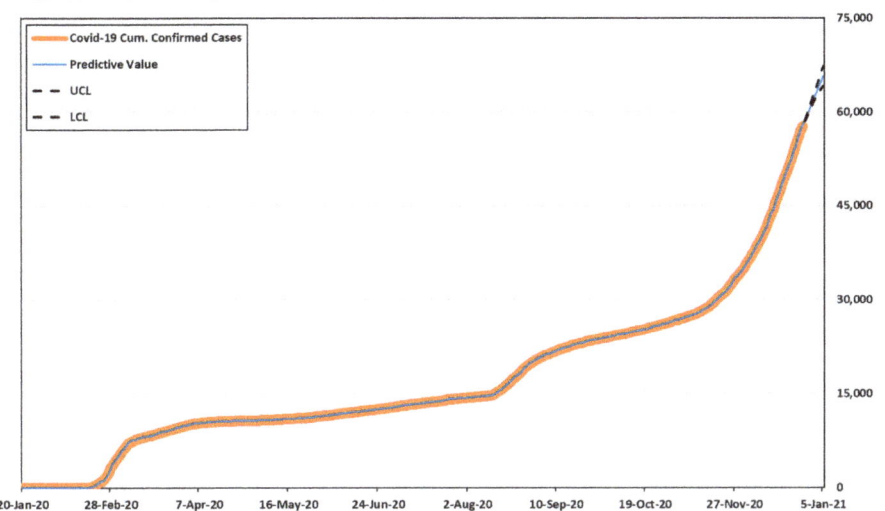

Figure 4. Time-series plot for the best ARIMA (1,2,5).

4. Discussion

In Section 3, we used ARIMA to compare the criteria of each case using data sets from Korea. The period between 20 January to 26 October 2020 was divided into five based on (1) peak of the first wave; (2) the day when the increase in confirmed cases is at its minimum; (3) the day when the variability of the confirmed case is high before the peak of the second wave; (4) peak of the second wave; and (5) the day when the variability of the confirmed cases is high before the peak of the third wave. Tables 3–7 show the top six results by comparing the goodness-of-fit of the ARIMA model for each group and case, and Table 8 shows the top five results based on SSE to examine the predicted values.

In general, if the goodness-of-fit is high, the predicted value is thought to be high, but the results were different. As can be seen from the note of the results in Table 8, the SSE value of the ARIMA model derived using ∆t 5 was significantly lower than that of other models.

It is recommended because it performs much better at predicting the number of confirmed cases using data at each point in time of the time interval 5, i.e., the average data of 5 days. By predicting the number of confirmed patients based on the results of analysis at various points in time using empirical data analysis and the ARIMA model using it, it is possible to preemptively respond to the variability (increase, decrease, rapid increase, etc.) of the number of confirmed patients through daily updates.

Additionally, in Korea, since the case definition is clear and data collection is almost in real time, the predictive power of the ARIMA model is relatively excellent and stable. There were unpredictable events due to the blind spot, but the blind spot is expected to gradually decrease due to the learning effect and preemptive examination on the similar exposure pathway. In addition, they successfully conducted a blind test as a way to cope with the phenomenon of avoiding tests due to social stigma, and there is a foundation for imposing legal sanctions in case of false reports on the route of infection. Prediction through the ARIMA model provides an important basis for KDCA to predict the necessary severe disease constant and prepare it in advance. In Korea, the proportion of public medical services is small, so the number of beds that can treat critically ill patients is limited. This is because it takes time to secure the number of severe illnesses by seeking cooperation from the private medical field. The accuracy of the prediction model is expected to improve as data is accumulated. However, there is a need for a model that can reflect the effects of external factors such as the effect of policy measures such as adjustment of the quarantine stage and the influx of mutant viruses.

5. Conclusions

This study aimed to suggest an appropriate prediction time point to significantly predict the number of confirmed cases. To significantly predict the number of confirmed COVID-19 cases in Korea, we proposed it should be analyzed and predicted using data at each point in time of the time interval 5, i.e., the average data of 5 days. Forecasting at this time can clearly confirm whether the number of cases will increase or decrease in the future.

The ARIMA model was fitted using the most recent data in progress for the third wave. As a result of predicting the number of cumulative confirmed cases for the next 14 days based on the best models of each criterion, the number of cumulative confirmed cases by the beginning of next year was expected to reach 70,000. Currently, Korea has a shortage of hospital beds. The results are expected to effectively estimate at the point the number of beds required by predicting variability (decrease and, increase) and the number of confirmed cases. In addition, this study is expected to help the government and Korea Disease Control and Prevention Agency (KDCA) to respond systematically to a future surge in confirmed cases.

However, it is difficult to accurately predict the changing cases, because various factors affect the increase in the number of confirmed cases. Furthermore, the influence of mass inflection is large. Therefore, it is necessary to study various techniques, such as reinforcement of machine learning, modeling research based on deep learning, and the application of prediction algorithms.

Author Contributions: D.H.L.: Formal analysis, Writing-Original Draft. Y.S.K.: Formal analysis, Software. Y.Y.K.: Writing—Review and Editing. K.Y.S.: Conceptualization, Writing—Original Draft, Writing—Review and Editing. I.H.C.: Writing—Review and Editing, Supervision, Funding acquisition. All authors have read and agreed to the published version of the manuscript.

Funding: This study was supported by research funds from Chosun University, 2020.

Institutional Review Board Statement: Not required.

Informed Consent Statement: Not applicable.

Data Availability Statement: Data available in a publicly accessible repository.

Acknowledgments: This study was supported by research funds from Chosun University, 2020.

Conflicts of Interest: The authors declare no conflict of interest.

References

1. World Economic Outlook: A Long and Difficult Ascent. Available online: https://www.imf.org/en/Publications/WEO/Issues/2020/09/30/world-economic-outlook-october-2020 (accessed on 12 October 2020).
2. Maliszewska, M.; Mattoo, A.; van der Mensbrugghe, D. The Potential Impact of COVID-19 on GDP and Trade: A Preliminary Assessment. *World Bank Policy Res. Work. Paper* **2020**. [CrossRef]
3. WHO Director-General's Opening Remarks at the Media Briefing on COVID-19—11 March 2020. Available online: https://www.who.int/director-general/speeches/detail/who-director-general-s-opening-remarks-at-the-media-briefing-on-covid-19---11-march-2020 (accessed on 11 December 2020).
4. Past Pandemics. Available online: https://www.cdc.gov/flu/pandemic-resources/basics/past-pandemics.html (accessed on 12 October 2020).
5. Johns Hopkins CSSE 'COVID19 Daily Reports'. Available online: https://www.arcgis.com/apps/opsdashboard/index.html#/bda7594740fd40299423467b48e9ecf6 (accessed on 11 December 2020).
6. Guan, P.; Huang, D.S.; Zhou, B. Sen Forecasting model for the incidence of hepatitis A based on artificial neural network. *World J. Gastroenterol.* **2004**, *10*, 3579–3582. [CrossRef]
7. Earnest, A.; Chen, M.I.; Ng, D.; Leo, Y.S. Using autoregressive integrated moving average (ARIMA) models to predict and monitor the number of beds occupied during a SARS outbreak in a tertiary hospital in Singapore. *BMC Health Serv. Res.* **2005**, *5*, 36. [CrossRef]
8. Liu, Q.; Liu, X.; Jiang, B.; Yang, W. Forecasting incidence of hemorrhagic fever with renal syndrome in China using ARIMA model. *BMC Infect. Dis.* **2011**, *11*, 218. [CrossRef] [PubMed]

9. Wu, W.; Guo, J.; An, S.; Guan, P.; Ren, Y.; Xia, L.; Zhou, B. Comparison of two hybrid models for forecasting the incidence of hemorrhagic fever with renal syndrome in Jiangsu Province, China. *PLoS ONE* **2015**, *10*, e0135492. [CrossRef] [PubMed]
10. Nsoesie, E.O.; Beckman, R.J.; Shashaani, S.; Nagaraj, K.S.; Marathe, M.V. A Simulation Optimization Approach to Epidemic Forecasting. *PLoS ONE* **2013**, *8*, e67164. [CrossRef]
11. Chen, Y.; Leng, K.; Lu, Y.; Wen, L.; Qi, Y.; Gao, W.; Chen, H.; Bai, L.; An, X.; Sun, B.; et al. Epidemiological features and time-series analysis of influenza incidence in urban and rural areas of Shenyang, China, 2010-2018. *Epidemiol. Infect.* **2020**, *148*, e29. [CrossRef]
12. Webb, G.; Magal, P.; Liu, Z.; Seydi, O. A model to predict COVID-19 epidemics with applications to South Korea, Italy, and Spain. *SIAM News* **2020**, *1*, 1–6. [CrossRef]
13. Alakus, T.B.; Turkoglu, I. Comparison of deep learning approaches to predict COVID-19 infection. *Chaos Solitons Fractals* **2020**, *140*. [CrossRef]
14. Pham, H. On estimating the number of deaths related to Covid-19. *Mathematics* **2020**, *8*, 655. [CrossRef]
15. Pham, H. Predictive modeling on the number of Covid-19 death toll in the united states considering the effects of coronavirus-related changes and Covid-19 recovered cases. *Int. J. Math. Eng. Manage. Sci.* **2020**, *5*, 1140–1155. [CrossRef]
16. Pham, H. Estimating the COVID-19 death toll by considering the time-dependent effects of various pandemic restrictions. *Mathematics* **2020**, *8*, 1628. [CrossRef]
17. Arias, V.; Alberto, M. Using generalized logistics regression to forecast population infected by Covid-19. *arXiv* **2020**, arXiv:2004.02406.
18. Kumar, P.; Singh, R.K.; Nanda, C.; Kalita, H.; Patairiya, S.; Sharma, Y.D.; Rani, M.; Bhagavathula, A.S. Forecasting COVID-19 impact in India using pandemic waves Nonlinear Growth Models. *MedRxiv* **2020**. [CrossRef]
19. Petropoulos, F.; Makridakis, S.; Stylianou, N. COVID-19: Forecasting confirmed cases and deaths with a simple time-series model. *Int. J. Forecast.* **2020**. [CrossRef]
20. Ceylan, Z. Estimation of COVID-19 prevalence in Italy, Spain, and France. *Sci. Total Environ.* **2020**, *729*, 133817. [CrossRef] [PubMed]
21. Alzahrani, S.I.; Aljamaan, I.A.; Al-Fakih, E.A. Forecasting the spread of the COVID-19 pandemic in Saudi Arabia using ARIMA prediction model under current public health interventions. *J. Infect. Public Health* **2020**, *13*, 914–919. [CrossRef]
22. Yang, Q.; Wang, J.; Ma, H.; Wang, X. Research on COVID-19 based on ARIMA modelΔ—Taking Hubei, China as an example to see the epidemic in Italy. *J. Infect. Public Health* **2020**, *13*, 1415–1418. [CrossRef]
23. Kufel, T. ARIMA-based forecasting of the dynamics of confirmed Covid-19 cases for selected European countries. *Equilibrium. Q. J. Econ. Econ. Policy* **2020**, *15*, 181–204. [CrossRef]
24. Benvenuto, D.; Giovanetti, M.; Vassallo, L.; Angeletti, S.; Ciccozzi, M. Application of the ARIMA model on the COVID-2019 epidemic dataset. *Data Br.* **2020**, *29*, 105340. [CrossRef] [PubMed]
25. Liu, Z.; Magal, P.; Webb, G. Predicting the number of reported and unreported cases for the COVID-19 epidemics in China, South Korea, Italy, France, Germany and United Kingdom. *J. Theor. Biol.* **2020**. [CrossRef] [PubMed]
26. Yang, S.; Cao, P.; Du, P.; Wu, Z.; Zhuang, Z.; Yang, L.; Yu, X.; Zhou, Q.; Feng, X.; Wang, X.; et al. Early estimation of the case fatality rate of COVID-19 in mainland China: A data-driven analysis. *Ann. Transl. Med.* **2020**, *8*, 128. [CrossRef]
27. Payne, J.L.; Morgan, A. COVID-19 and Violent Crime: A comparison of recorded offence rates and dynamic forecasts (ARIMA) for March 2020 in Queensland, Australia. *Preprint* **2020**. [CrossRef]
28. Matthew, E.; Adeyinka, O. Application of Hierarchical Polynomial Regression Models to Predict Transmission of COVID-19 at Global Level. *Int. J. Clin. Biostat. Biom.* **2020**, *6*. [CrossRef]
29. Ilie, O.D.; Cojocariu, R.O.; Ciobica, A.; Timofte, S.I.; Mavroudis, I.; Doroftei, B. Forecasting the spreading of COVID-19 across nine countries from Europe, Asia, and the American continents using the arima models. *Microorganisms* **2020**, *8*, 1158. [CrossRef] [PubMed]
30. Song, J.-Y.; Yun, J.-G.; Noh, J.-Y.; Cheong, H.-J.; Kim, W.-J. Covid-19 in South Korea—Challenges of Subclinical Manifestations. *N. Engl. J. Med.* **2020**, *382*, 1858–1859. [CrossRef]
31. Cases in Korea. Available online: http://ncov.mohw.go.kr/en/bdBoardList.do?brdId=16&brdGubun=161&dataGubun=&ncvContSeq=&contSeq=&board_id= (accessed on 12 October 2020).
32. Protestant Churches under Fire for Holding Sunday Services Despite Coronavirus Epidemic. Available online: http://news.koreaherald.com/view.php?ud=20200317000794&ACE_SEARCH=1 (accessed on 12 October 2020).
33. Korea Reports 323 New COVID-19 Cases. Available online: http://news.koreaherald.com/view.php?ud=20200829000051&ACE_SEARCH=1 (accessed on 12 October 2020).
34. COVID-19 Cases See Largest Daily Increase since August. Available online: Ttp://news.koreaherald.com/view.php?ud=20201125000190&ACE_SEARCH=1 (accessed on 11 December 2020).
35. Box, G.E.; Jenkins, G.M.; Reinsel, G.C.; Ljung, G.M. *Time Series Analysis: Forecasting and Control*, 4th ed.; John Wiley & Sons: Hoboken, NJ, USA, 2015; ISBN 9781118674925.

MDPI
St. Alban-Anlage 66
4052 Basel
Switzerland
Tel. +41 61 683 77 34
Fax +41 61 302 89 18
www.mdpi.com

Healthcare Editorial Office
E-mail: healthcare@mdpi.com
www.mdpi.com/journal/healthcare

www.ingramcontent.com/pod-product-compliance
Lightning Source LLC
LaVergne TN
LVHW070631100526
838202LV00012B/777